CIRRHOSIS OF THE LIVER COOKBOOK

Learn how to prepare easy, quick, delicious friendly recipes to improve your liver wellbeing with 14-day meal plan

Bonus: meal planner journal

By

Ben Georg

Copyright © Ben Georg

All right reserved

No part of book may be reproduced or stored in a retrieval system or transmitted in any form or by any means, electronic, mechanical, photocopying, recording or otherwise, without express written permission of the publisher

Thanks for your purchase

You are our voice without you we don't exist, kindly help leave an honest review on amazon.

Would you like to check out my other books on health and diet?

SCAN THE QRCODE BELOW IT WILL LEAD YOU MY AUTHOR CENTRAL ON AMAZON.

Content

INTRODUCTION

Welcome to the "Cirrhosis of the Liver Cookbook," a comprehensive guide designed to support individuals navigating the challenges of liver cirrhosis through a thoughtful approach to nutrition. Living with cirrhosis requires special attention to diet and lifestyle, and this cookbook aims to provide not just recipes but a wealth of information to empower individuals in managing their condition effectively.

Cirrhosis is a serious liver condition that demands a nuanced approach to dietary choices. Whether you are personally affected or supporting a loved one, understanding the impact of nutrition on liver health is crucial. In this cookbook, we delve into the intricacies of cirrhosis, exploring its causes, risk factors, and preventive measures. By gaining insight into the condition, you can make informed choices to enhance your well-being.

The heart of this cookbook lies in the section dedicated to a liver cirrhosis diet. We explore the foods that are beneficial and those that should be limited or avoided. Our goal is to offer a variety of delicious and nourishing recipes that align with the dietary recommendations for individuals managing cirrhosis. Each recipe is crafted not only for its taste but also with a focus on supporting liver health.

As we embark on this culinary journey together, let this cookbook be a trusted companion on your path to better nutrition and overall well-being. May these recipes not only tantalize your taste buds but also contribute to the overall management of cirrhosis, fostering a sense of control and vitality in your daily life. Cheers to delicious and health-conscious cooking!

Liver cirrhosis is a chronic and progressive condition characterized by the scarring of liver tissue. This scarring, also known as fibrosis disrupts the normal structure of the liver and hinders its vital functions. The liver, a resilient organ with remarkable regenerative capabilities, can sustain damage over time due to various factors, leading to the development of cirrhosis.

One of the primary roles of the liver is to process nutrients, filter toxins from the blood, and produce proteins necessary for blood clotting. When cirrhosis occurs, the liver's ability to perform these functions is compromised. Scar tissue replaces healthy liver cells, impairing blood flow through the organ and disrupting its normal processes.

Understanding the progression of cirrhosis involves recognizing the four stages of the condition. In the initial stages, the liver may still function relatively well despite the presence of some scarring. However, as cirrhosis advances, the liver's capacity to perform essential functions diminishes, ultimately leading to liver failure.

Common causes of liver cirrhosis include chronic alcohol consumption, viral hepatitis infections (such as hepatitis B and C), non-alcoholic fatty liver disease (NAFLD), autoimmune liver diseases, and certain genetic disorders. Additionally, prolonged exposure to certain toxins and medications can contribute to liver damage and cirrhosis.

The symptoms of liver cirrhosis can vary, and some individuals may not exhibit noticeable signs until the disease has progressed. Symptoms may include fatigue, weakness, abdominal swelling, easy bruising, and confusion. It is crucial for individuals at risk or experiencing symptoms to seek medical attention for proper diagnosis and management.

By understanding the complexities of liver cirrhosis, individuals can make informed decisions about their lifestyle, including dietary choices, and work closely with healthcare professionals to manage the condition effectively. Early detection, lifestyle modifications, and appropriate medical care play crucial roles in improving outcomes for individuals with liver cirrhosis.

Cirrhosis is a serious and irreversible condition, but several proactive measures can significantly reduce the risk of its development. Adopting a lifestyle focused on liver health can be instrumental in preventing the progression of liver disease. Here are key strategies for the prevention of cirrhosis:

1. **Moderate Alcohol Consumption:** Excessive alcohol intake is a leading cause of cirrhosis. To protect the liver, it is essential to limit alcohol consumption. Moderation is key, and for those with a history of liver disease or other risk factors, complete abstinence may be recommended.

2. **Vaccination Against Hepatitis:** Certain types of viral hepatitis, particularly hepatitis B and C, can lead to cirrhosis. Ensuring vaccination against hepatitis and practicing safe behaviors to prevent infection are crucial preventive measures.

3. **Maintain a Healthy Weight:** Non-alcoholic fatty liver disease (NAFLD) is a common precursor to cirrhosis. Maintaining a healthy weight through a balanced diet and regular exercise can help prevent the accumulation of fat in the liver.

4. **Manage Chronic Conditions:** Conditions such as diabetes and high blood pressure can contribute to liver damage. Effective management of these chronic conditions through medication, lifestyle changes, and regular medical check-ups can reduce the risk of cirrhosis.

5. **Avoid Hepatotoxic Substances:** Exposure to certain toxins and chemicals can harm the liver. It is crucial to minimize contact with hepatotoxic substances, whether they are environmental toxins or specific medications that may pose a risk to liver health.

6. **Practice Safe Sex:** Sexual transmission of hepatitis can occur. Practicing safe sex and using protective measures can reduce the risk of contracting and spreading hepatitis viruses.

7. **Regular Medical Check-ups:** Routine medical check-ups, especially for individuals with known risk factors, can facilitate early detection and intervention. Regular monitoring of liver function through blood tests and imaging studies can identify issues before they progress to cirrhosis.

8. **Healthy Dietary Choices:** A balanced and nutritious diet plays a crucial role in liver health. Limiting the intake of

processed foods, saturated fats, and sugars while increasing consumption of fruits, vegetables, and whole grains supports overall well-being and liver function.

9. **Stay Hydrated:** Proper hydration is essential for liver function. Drinking an adequate amount of water helps the liver flush out toxins and supports overall metabolic processes.

10. **Educate and Raise Awareness:** Public awareness campaigns can contribute to the prevention of cirrhosis by educating individuals about the risks and promoting healthy lifestyle choices.

By incorporating these preventive measures into one's lifestyle and seeking professional guidance when needed, individuals can take significant steps to reduce the risk of cirrhosis and promote long-term liver health.

CAUSE AND RISK FACTOR OF THE CIRRHOSIS OF THE LIVER

Cirrhosis of the liver can result from various factors, each contributing to the gradual scarring and impairment of the liver's function. Understanding the causes and risk factors is essential for prevention and early intervention. Here are some key contributors to the development of cirrhosis:

1. **Chronic Alcohol Consumption:** One of the primary causes of cirrhosis is chronic alcohol abuse. Prolonged and excessive alcohol intake can lead to inflammation, fatty liver disease, and ultimately, cirrhosis.

2. **Viral Hepatitis Infections:** Hepatitis B and C viruses pose a significant risk for cirrhosis. These infections can lead to chronic inflammation of the liver, causing progressive damage over time.

3. **Non-Alcoholic Fatty Liver Disease (NAFLD):** NAFLD is characterized by the accumulation of fat in the liver, often associated with obesity, insulin resistance, and metabolic syndrome. If left unaddressed, NAFLD can progress to cirrhosis.

4. **Autoimmune Liver Diseases:** Conditions such as autoimmune hepatitis, primary biliary cholangitis, and primary sclerosing cholangitis involve the immune system mistakenly attacking liver cells, leading to inflammation and scarring.

5. **Genetic Disorders:** Certain genetic conditions, such as hemochromatosis, Wilson's disease, and alpha-1 antitrypsin deficiency, can predispose individuals to cirrhosis by

affecting the liver's ability to process and store essential substances.

6. **Chronic Hepatotoxic Medications:** Long-term use of certain medications, especially those with hepatotoxic properties, can contribute to liver damage and cirrhosis. Regular monitoring and consultation with healthcare professionals are crucial for those on such medications.

7. **Biliary Tract Disorders:** Conditions affecting the bile ducts, such as biliary atresia or repeated episodes of gallstone obstruction, can lead to cirrhosis by impairing the normal flow of bile.

8. **Cystic Fibrosis:** Individuals with cystic fibrosis may develop cirrhosis due to complications affecting the pancreas and liver.

9. **Metabolic Disorders:** Disorders like glycogen storage diseases and Alagille syndrome can disrupt normal metabolic processes, impacting the liver and potentially leading to cirrhosis.

10. **Prolonged Exposure to Toxins:** Occupational exposure to certain toxins and chemicals, as well as environmental pollutants, can contribute to liver damage and cirrhosis over time.

11. **Age and Gender:** Cirrhosis tends to be more prevalent in older individuals, and men are often at a higher risk compared to women. However, the risk can vary based on individual health and lifestyle factors.

Recognizing these causes and risk factors enables individuals and healthcare professionals to identify those at higher risk for cirrhosis and implement preventive measures. Early intervention and management of underlying conditions can significantly reduce the likelihood of cirrhosis development. Regular health check-ups and a proactive approach to liver health are essential components of minimizing risk.

How to follow a liver cirrhosis diet

Adopting a liver-friendly diet is a crucial aspect of managing cirrhosis and supporting overall liver health. The following list outlines foods that are generally considered beneficial for individuals with cirrhosis:

1. **Lean Protein Sources:**

   - Skinless poultry

   - Fish (especially fatty fish like salmon, mackerel, and sardines)

   - Lean cuts of meat

   - Eggs (in moderation)

2. **Low-Fat Dairy:**

   - Skim or low-fat milk

   - Greek yogurt

   - Cottage cheese

3. **Fruits:**

   - Fresh fruits (such as apples, berries, and citrus fruits)

   - Dried fruits (in moderation)

4. **Vegetables:**

   - Leafy greens (spinach, kale, and collard greens)

   - Cruciferous vegetables (broccoli, cauliflower)

- Colorful vegetables (carrots, bell peppers)

5. **Whole Grains:**

   - Quinoa

   - Brown rice

   - Oats

   - Whole wheat products (bread, pasta)

6. **Healthy Fats:**

   - Olive oil

   - Avocado

   - Nuts and seeds (in moderation)

7. **Fluids:**

   - Water is essential for hydration and supports overall liver function.

   - Herbal teas (without caffeine)

   - Fresh fruit juices (in moderation)

8. **Limited Sodium Intake:**

   - Minimize salt intake to help manage fluid retention.

   - Use herbs and spices for flavor instead of salt.

9. **Small, Frequent Meals:**

   - Consuming smaller, more frequent meals rather than large meals can help ease the workload on the liver.

10. **Supplements (Under Medical Guidance):**

- Depending on individual needs, healthcare professionals may recommend specific supplements such as vitamin D, vitamin B complex, and others.

It's important for individuals with cirrhosis to tailor their diet to their specific needs and consult with healthcare professionals or a registered dietitian. While these food choices are generally considered beneficial, individual tolerance and preferences can vary. Monitoring nutritional status and making adjustments based on any dietary restrictions or symptoms is crucial for optimal liver health. Always seek personalized advice from healthcare providers for a diet plan that suits individual health conditions and requirements.

Managing cirrhosis involves not only incorporating beneficial foods but also avoiding certain items that can exacerbate liver damage and hinder overall health. Here's a list of foods that individuals with cirrhosis are typically advised to limit or avoid:

1. **High-Sodium Foods:**

   - Processed and packaged foods

   - Canned soups and broths

   - Salty snacks (chips, pretzels)

2. **Fried and Fatty Foods:**

   - Deep-fried items

   - Fast food

   - Fatty cuts of meat

   - Full-fat dairy products

3. **Red and Processed Meats:**

   - Beef, pork, and lamb (especially processed varieties)

   - Sausages and hot dogs

4. **High-Sugar Foods:**

   - Sugary snacks and desserts

   - Sweetened beverages (sodas, energy drinks)

   - Candies and pastries

5. **Excessive Alcohol:**

- Alcohol is a significant contributor to liver damage, and complete abstinence is often recommended for individuals with cirrhosis.

6. **High-Protein Diets (Under Medical Guidance):**

   - While protein is essential, excessive intake may stress the liver. Consult with healthcare professionals to determine the appropriate protein level for individual needs.

7. **Caffeine in Excess:**

   - While moderate consumption of caffeine is generally considered safe, excessive intake may have adverse effects on liver health.

8. **High-Oxalate Foods (For Those with Liver Disease-Related Kidney Issues):**

   - Spinach, beets, nuts, and certain other high-oxalate foods should be limited for individuals with kidney complications associated with liver disease.

9. **Raw Seafood:**

   - Raw or undercooked seafood, such as oysters and sushi, may pose a risk of infection, especially in individuals with compromised liver function.

10. **Certain Herbal Supplements (Without Medical Approval):**

    - Some herbal supplements may interact with medications or affect liver function. Always consult with healthcare professionals before incorporating herbal remedies.

11. **Large Meals:**

- Consuming large meals can strain the liver. Opt for smaller, more frequent meals to ease the workload on the digestive system.

It's crucial for individuals with cirrhosis to work closely with healthcare professionals, including dietitians, to tailor dietary recommendations to their specific needs. While this list provides general guidance, individual tolerances and dietary restrictions can vary. Regular monitoring of nutritional status and adjustments to the diet based on medical advice are essential for supporting liver health and overall well-being.

4 STAGES IF CIRRHOSIS OF THE LIVER

The progression of cirrhosis of the liver is commonly classified into four stages, each representing a different level of severity and impact on liver function. These stages help healthcare professionals assess the extent of liver damage and determine appropriate interventions. The four stages of cirrhosis are:

1. **Compensated Cirrhosis (Stage 1 and 2):**

   - In the early stages, the liver may still be able to function relatively well despite the presence of some scarring (fibrosis).

   - Symptoms may be minimal or absent, and individuals may not be aware of the underlying liver condition.

   - Liver function tests may show abnormalities, but the damage is not yet significantly affecting day-to-day activities.

- At this point, lifestyle changes and management of underlying causes may slow or halt the progression of cirrhosis.

2. **Decompensated Cirrhosis (Stage 3):**

   - As cirrhosis progresses, the liver's ability to perform essential functions becomes compromised.

   - Symptoms become more noticeable and may include fatigue, weakness, easy bruising, and fluid retention (edema and ascites).

   - Decompensated cirrhosis indicates a significant loss of liver function, leading to complications that may require medical intervention.

3. **Advanced Cirrhosis (Stage 4):**

   - Also known as end-stage cirrhosis or decompensated cirrhosis with complications.

   - Severe scarring has occurred, severely impairing liver function.

   - Symptoms become more severe, and complications such as hepatic encephalopathy (confusion and cognitive dysfunction) and bleeding from varices may occur.

   - Liver transplant evaluation may be considered for eligible candidates at this stage.

4. **Liver Failure (End-Stage):**

   - This stage represents a critical condition where the liver is unable to perform its essential functions adequately.

- Symptoms escalate, and life-threatening complications, such as kidney failure, severe bleeding, and infection, may arise.

- Liver transplantation is often the only definitive treatment option for end-stage liver failure.

It's important to note that the progression of cirrhosis can vary from person to person, and not everyone with cirrhosis will experience all stages. Regular monitoring through medical check-ups, liver function tests, and imaging studies helps healthcare professionals assess the stage of cirrhosis and tailor appropriate management strategies. Early detection and intervention in the earlier stages can improve outcomes and potentially slow or halt the progression of the condition. Individuals diagnosed with cirrhosis should work closely with healthcare providers to develop a comprehensive care plan based on their specific needs.

Cirrhosis Recipes

1. Tomato Scrambled Eggs with

Feta Cheese

Ingredients:

- 1/4 cup olive oil

- 2 Roma tomatoes, chopped

- 1/4 cup minced red onion

- 2 garlic cloves, minced

- 1/2 tsp dried oregano

- 1/2 tsp dried thyme

- 8 large eggs

- 3/4 cup feta cheese, crumbled

- 1/4 cup fresh cilantro, chopped

- Salt & black pepper to taste

Directions:

1. In a big skillet over medium heat, warm the olive oil. When the tomatoes are tender, add the chopped tomatoes and red onion and sauté for ten minutes.

2. Add the minced garlic, oregano, and thyme, continuing to sauté for an additional 1-2 minutes until the liquid reduces.

3. Combine the eggs, salt, and pepper in a medium-sized bowl and whisk until thoroughly mixed.

4. Remove the skillet from heat, stir in the crumbled feta and chopped cilantro, and serve.

Nutrition Information:

Calories: 338

Fat: 8g

Carbs: 6g

Protein: 16g

Prep time: 10

Cooking time: 16

Serving 4

2. Morning Baklava French toast

Ingredients:

• 2 tbsp orange juice

• 3 fresh eggs, beaten

• 1 tsp lemon zest

• 1/8 tsp vanilla extract

• ¼ cup honey

• 2 tbsp almond milk

• ¾ tsp ground cinnamon

• ¼ cup walnuts, crumbled

• ¼ cup pistachios, crumbled

• 1 tbsp sugar

• 2 tbsp white bread crumbs

• 4 slices bread

• 2 tbsp unsalted butter

• 1 tsp confectioners' sugar

Directions:

1. Combine the eggs, orange juice, lemon

zest, vanilla, honey, milk, and cinnamon

in a bowl; set aside. Pulse walnuts and

pistachios in a food processor until they

are finely crumbled.

2. In a small bowl, mix the walnuts, pistachios, sugar, and bread crumbs. Spread the nut mixture on 2 bread slices.

3. Cover with the remaining 2 slices. Melt the butter in a skillet over medium heat. Dip the sandwiches into the egg mixture and fry them for 4 minutes on both sides or until golden.

4. Remove to a plate and cut them diagonally. Dust with confectioners' sugar. Serve immediately.

Nutrition: Calories: 651; Fat: 7g; Carbs: 80g; Protein: 21g

CIRRHOSIS CO

Prep time: 10

Cooking time: 4

Serving 4

3. Buckwheat Porridge

Ingredients:

- 3 cups water

- 2 cups raw buckwheat groats

- Pinch of sea salt

- 1 cup unsweetened almond milk

Directions:

1. Place the water, sea salt, and buckwheat groats in a medium saucepan. Heat the mixture on medium-high and bring it to a boil.

2. Turn down the heat after it starts to boil. Cook, stirring periodically, until most of the water is absorbed, about 20 minutes.

3. Completely whisk in the unsweetened almond milk after folding it in. Cook the buckwheat groats for a further 15 minutes or until they are tender. Spoon the oatmeal into dishes and reheat.

Nutrition Information:

Calories: 121

Fat: 1.0g

Carbs: 21.5g

Protein: 6.3g

Prep time: 10

Cooking time: 35

Serving 4

4. Egg in a "Pepper Hole" with Avocado

Ingredients:

- 4 bell peppers, any color, stemmed and seeded, with 2 peppers cut into 2-inch-thick rings and the rest chopped

- 1 tablespoon extra-virgin olive oil

- 8 large eggs

- 3/4 teaspoon kosher salt, divided

- 1/4 teaspoon freshly ground black pepper, divided

- 1 avocado, peeled, pitted, and diced

- 1/4 cup red onion, diced

- 1/4 cup fresh basil, chopped

- Juice of 1/2 lime

Directions:

1. In a big skillet over medium heat, warm the olive oil. Place one egg in the center of each of the four bell pepper rings after adding them. Add 1/8 teaspoon black pepper and 1/4 teaspoon salt for seasoning.

2. Cook for 2 to 3 minutes until the egg whites are mostly set but the yolks are still runny. Gently flip and cook for an additional minute for over easy.

3. Transfer the egg-bell pepper rings to a platter or onto plates, and repeat the process with the remaining 4 bell pepper rings.

4. In a medium bowl, combine the avocado, onion, basil, lime juice, reserved diced bell pepper, the remaining 1/4 teaspoon

kosher salt, and remaining black pepper. Serve over the cooked egg-bell pepper rings.

Nutrition Information:

Calories: 270

Fat: 9g

Carbs: 12g

Protein: 15g

Prep time: 10min

Cooking time: 4-5 min

Serving 4

5. Avocado Toast with Smoked Trout

Ingredients:

- 1 avocado, peeled and pitted

- 2 teaspoons lemon juice, plus extra for serving

- 3/4 teaspoon ground cumin

- 1/4 teaspoon kosher salt

- 1/4 teaspoon red pepper flakes, plus extra for sprinkling

- 1/4 teaspoon lemon zest

- 2 slices whole-wheat bread, toasted

- 1 (3.75-ounce) can of smoked trout

Directions:

1. In a medium bowl, mash together the avocado, lemon juice, cumin, salt, red pepper flakes, and lemon zest.

2. Top each slice of toast with half of the avocado mixture. Place half of the smoked fish on top of each piece of toast.

3. Garnish with a pinch of red pepper flakes (if desired) and/or a sprinkle of lemon juice (if desired).

Nutrition Information:

Calories: 300

Fat: 4g

Carbs: 21g

Protein: 11g

Prep time: 10

Cooking time:0

Serving 2

6. Kale Egg Cups

Ingredients:

- 1 slice of whole-grain bread

- 4 large eggs, beaten

- 3 tablespoons milk

- 1/2 teaspoon onion powder

- 1/4 teaspoon garlic powder

- 3/4 cup chopped kale

- Salt and black pepper to taste

Directions:

1. Preheat the oven to 350°F. Break the whole-grain bread into pieces and distribute them evenly between two greased ramekins.

2. In a medium bowl, combine the beaten eggs, milk, salt, onion powder, garlic powder, pepper, and chopped kale. Mix well.

3. Pour half of the egg mixture into each ramekin and bake for 25 minutes or until the eggs are set.

4. Serve and enjoy this nutritious baked kale and egg dish!

Nutrition Information:

Calories: 213

Fat: 12g

Carbs: 13g

Protein: 17g

Prep time: 10

Cooking time: 25

Serving 2

7. Banana Pancakes With Strawberries

Ingredients:

- 2 tablespoons olive oil

- 1 cup almond flour

- 1 cup + 2 tablespoons almond milk

- 2 beaten eggs

- 1/3 cup honey

- 1 teaspoon baking soda

- 1/4 teaspoon salt

- 1 sliced banana

- 1 cup sliced strawberries

- 1 tablespoon maple syrup

Directions:

1. In a bowl, combine almond flour, almond milk, beaten eggs, honey, baking soda, and salt. Mix thoroughly.

2. Warm olive oil in a skillet over medium heat. Pour 1/3 cup of batter and cook for 2-3 minutes.

3. Add half of the sliced fresh fruit, flip, and cook for an additional 2-3 minutes until cooked through.

4. Top the pancakes with the remaining fruit, drizzle with maple syrup, and serve.

Nutrition Information:

Calories: 415

Fat: 4g

Carbs: 46g

Protein: 12g

Prep time: 10 cooking time: 6 serving 4

8. Pecan & Peach Parfait

Ingredients:

- 1 1/2 cups plain low-fat yogurt

- 1/2 cup pecans

- 1/2 cup whole-grain rolled oats

- 1 teaspoon honey

- 1 peach, peeled and chopped

- Mint leaves for garnish

Directions:

1. Preheat your oven to 310°F. Spread the oats and pecans evenly on a baking sheet. Toast for 11-13 minutes, then set aside.

2. Microwave the honey for 30 seconds, and mix it with the chopped peach.

3. In 2 glasses, layer some of the peach mixture, followed by yogurt, and sprinkle with the toasted oat mixture.

4. Repeat the layering process until all the ingredients are used, finishing with the peach mixture on top. Garnish with mint leaves.

Nutrition Information:

Calories: 403

Fat: 9g

Carbs: 40g

Protein: 22g

Prep time: 10 cooking time: 14 serving 2

9. Breakfast Pita Sandwiches
 Ingredients:

- 2 eggs, boiled, peeled, and sliced

- 1 small avocado, peeled, halved, and pitted

- 1 (8-inch) whole-wheat pocket pita bread, halved

- 12 (1/4-inch) thick cucumber slices

- 6 oil-packed sun-dried tomatoes, rinsed, patted dry, and cut in half

- 2 tablespoons crumbled feta

- 1/2 teaspoon extra virgin olive oil

- 1/4 teaspoon fresh lemon juice

- 1/4 teaspoon freshly ground black pepper

- Pinch of salt

Directions:

1. Use a fork to mash the avocado in a small bowl. Add lemon juice and salt, mash to combine, and spread half of the avocado mixture over one side of the pita half.

2. Sprinkle black pepper over the egg slices. Top the pita half with one sliced egg, 6 cucumber slices, and 6 sun-dried tomato pieces.

3. Sprinkle 1 tablespoon crumbled feta over the top and drizzle 1/4 teaspoon olive oil over the feta. Repeat with the other pita half. Serve promptly.

Nutrition Information:

Calories: 427

Fat: 8g

Carbs: 36g

Protein: 14g

Prep time: 15 cooking time: 0 serving 2

10. Chia & Almond Oatmeal
Ingredients:

- 1/4 teaspoon almond extract

- 1/2 cup milk

- 1/2 cup rolled oats

- 2 tablespoons sliced almonds

- 2 tablespoons sugar

- 1 teaspoon chia seeds

- 1/4 teaspoon ground cardamom

- 1/4 teaspoon ground cinnamon

Directions:

1. In a mason jar, combine milk, oats, almonds, sugar, chia seeds, cardamom, almond extract, and cinnamon. Shake the jar well to mix the ingredients.

2. Refrigerate the mixture for 4 hours. Serve and enjoy!

Nutrition Information:

Calories: 131

Fat: 6.2g

Carbs: 17g

Protein: 4.9g

Prep time: 15 cooking time: 0 serving 2

11. Breakfast Bulgur with Berries

Ingredients:

- 1/2 cup medium-grain bulgur wheat

- 1 cup water

- 1/4 cup unsweetened almond milk

- 1 teaspoon pure vanilla extract

- 1/4 teaspoon ground cinnamon

- 1 cup fresh berries of your choice

- Pinch of sea salt

Directions:

1. In a medium saucepan, combine bulgur with water and a pinch of sea salt, bringing it to a boil.

2. Cover the saucepan, remove it from heat, and let it stand for 10 minutes until the water is absorbed.

3. Stir in the almond milk, vanilla extract, and ground cinnamon until fully incorporated. Divide the mixture between two bowls and top with fresh berries to serve.

Nutrition Information:

Calories: 173

Fat: 1.6g

Carbs: 34.0g

Protein: 5.7g

Prep time: 10

Cooking time: 5

Serving 2

12. Strawberry Basil Honey Ricotta

Toast

Ingredients:

- 4 slices of toasted whole-grain bread

- 1/2 cup ricotta cheese

- 1 tablespoon honey

- 1 cup fresh strawberries, sliced

- 4 large fresh basil leaves, thinly sliced

- Sea salt to taste

Directions:

1. In a small bowl, combine the ricotta, honey, and a pinch or two of sea salt. Taste and adjust with additional honey or salt if desired.

2. Spread the ricotta mixture evenly over each slice of bread (about 2 tablespoons per slice).

3. Top each piece with sliced strawberries and a few pieces of shredded basil.

Nutrition Information:

Calories: 275

Fat: 8g

Carbs: 41g

Protein: 15g

Prep time: 10

Cooking time: 0

Serving 2

13. Parsley Tomato Eggs

Ingredients:

- 2 tablespoons olive oil

- 1 onion, chopped

- 2 garlic cloves, minced

- 2 cans diced tomatoes

- 6 large eggs

- 1/2 cup fresh chives, chopped

Directions:

1. In a large skillet over medium heat, heat the olive oil. Add the chopped onion and minced garlic, cooking for 3 minutes and stirring occasionally.

2. Pour in the diced tomatoes with their juices, and cook for an additional 3 minutes until the mixture is bubbling.

3. Crack one egg into a small custard cup. Using a large spoon, create six indentations in the tomato mixture.

4. Gently pour the first cracked egg into one indentation and repeat the process, cracking the remaining eggs one at a time into the custard cup and pouring one into each indentation.

5. Cover the skillet and cook for 6-8 minutes. Top with chopped chives and serve.

Nutrition Information:

Calories: 123

Fat: 8g

Carbs: 4g

Protein: 7g

Prep time: 10

Cooking time: 12-15

Serving 6

14. Garlic Bell Pepper Omelet

Ingredients:

- 2 tablespoons olive oil

- 2 red bell peppers, chopped

- 1/4 teaspoon nutmeg

- 4 eggs, beaten

- 2 garlic cloves, crushed

- 1 teaspoon Italian seasoning

Directions:

1. In a skillet over medium heat, warm the olive oil. Stir-fry the chopped red bell peppers for 3 minutes or until they are lightly charred; set them aside. Add the crushed garlic to the skillet and sauté for 1 minute.

2. Pour the beaten eggs over the garlic, sprinkle with Italian seasoning and nutmeg, and cook for 2-3 minutes or until the eggs are set.

3. Using a spatula, loosen the edges of the cooked eggs and gently slide them onto a plate. Add the charred peppers, fold over, and serve hot.

Nutrition Information:

Calories: 272

Fat: 12g

Carbs: 6.4g

Protein: 12g

Prep time: 10

Cooking time: 7

Serving 2

1. Pesto-Glazed Chicken Breasts

Preparation Time: 10 minutes

Cooking Time: 20 minutes

Servings: 4

Ingredients:

- 1/4 cup + 1 tablespoon extra-virgin olive oil, divided

- 4 boneless, skinless chicken breasts

- 1/2 teaspoon salt

- 1/4 teaspoon freshly ground black pepper

- 1 cup packed fresh basil leaves

- 1 garlic clove, minced

- 1/4 cup grated Parmesan cheese

- 1/4 cup pine nuts

Directions:

1. In a large, heavy skillet, heat 1 tablespoon of olive oil over medium-high heat.

2. Season the chicken breasts on both sides with salt and pepper, then place them in the skillet.

3. Cook for 10 minutes, flip, and cook for an additional 5 minutes.

4. Meanwhile, in a blender or food processor, combine the basil, garlic, Parmesan cheese, and pine nuts. Blend on high.

5. Gradually pour in the remaining 1/4 cup of olive oil and blend until smooth.

6. Spread 1 tablespoon of pesto on each chicken breast, cover the skillet, and cook for 5 minutes. Serve the chicken with the pesto side up.

Nutrition Information:

Calories: 531

Fat: 8g

Carbs: 2g

Protein: 64g

2. Arugula Spinach Salad with Shaved Parmesan

Prep time: 10 minutes

Cooking Time: 2 minutes

Servings: 3

Ingredients:

- 3 tablespoons raw pine nuts

- 3 cups arugula

- 3 cups baby leaf spinach

- 5 dried figs, pitted and chopped

- 2 1/2 ounces shaved Parmesan cheese

For the Dressing:

- 4 teaspoons balsamic vinegar

- 1 teaspoon low-sodium Dijon mustard

- 1 teaspoon honey

- 5 tablespoons extra virgin olive oil

Directions:

1. In a small pan over low heat, toast the pine nuts for 2 minutes or until they begin to brown. Remove promptly from the heat and transfer to a small bowl.

2. Make the dressing by combining balsamic vinegar, Dijon mustard, and honey in a small bowl. Use a fork to whisk, gradually adding the olive oil while continuously mixing.

3. In a large bowl, toss the arugula and baby spinach, then top with the figs, Parmesan cheese, and toasted pine nuts.

4. Drizzle the dressing over the top and toss until the ingredients are thoroughly coated. Serve promptly.

Nutrition Information:

Calories: 416

Fat: 5g

Carbs: 18g

Protein: 10g

3. Shrimp Quinoa Bowl with Black Olives

Preparation Time: 10 minutes

Cooking Time: 15 minutes

Servings: 4

Ingredients:

- 10 black olives, pitted and halved

- 1/4 cup olive oil

- 1 cup quinoa

- 1 lemon, cut into wedges

- 1 pound shrimp, peeled and cooked

- 2 tomatoes, sliced

- 2 bell peppers, thinly sliced

- 1 red onion, chopped

- 1 teaspoon dried dill

- 1 tablespoon fresh parsley, chopped

- Salt and black pepper to taste

Directions:

1. Place the quinoa in a pot and cover it with 2 cups of water over medium heat. Allow it to boil, then reduce the heat and simmer for 12-15 minutes until tender.

2. Take the quinoa off the stove and use a fork to fluff it up. Stir in the black pepper, dill, and parsley along with the olive oil.

3. Stir in the tomatoes, bell peppers, olives, and onion. Serve the bowl decorated with shrimp and lemon wedges.

Nutrition Information:

Calories: 362

Fat: 11g

Carbs: 38g

Protein: 79g

4. Margherita Open-Face Sandwiches

Preparation Time: 10 minutes

Cooking Time: 2 minutes

Servings: 4

Ingredients:

- 2 (6- to 7-inch) whole-wheat submarine or hoagie rolls, sliced open horizontally

- 1 tablespoon extra-virgin olive oil

- 1 garlic clove, halved

- 1 large ripe tomato, cut into 8 slices

- 1/4 teaspoon dried oregano

- 1 cup fresh mozzarella (about 4 oz), patted dry and sliced

- 1/4 cup lightly packed fresh basil leaves, torn into small pieces

- 1/4 teaspoon freshly ground black pepper

Directions:

1. Preheat the broiler to high with the rack 4 inches under the heating element.

2. Place the sliced bread on a large, rimmed baking sheet. Put it under the broiler for 1 minute, until the bread is lightly toasted. Remove from the oven.

3. Brush each piece of the toasted bread with the oil, and rub a garlic half over each piece.

4. Place the toasted bread back on the baking sheet. Evenly distribute the tomato slices on each piece, sprinkle with oregano, and layer the cheese on top.

5. Place the baking sheet under the broiler. Set the timer for 1.5 minutes, but check after 1 minute.

6. Remove the sandwiches, top each with fresh basil and pepper.

Nutrition Information:

Calories: 176

Fat: 9g

Carbs: 14g

Protein: 10g

5. Zucchini with Bow Ties

Preparation Time: 10 minutes

Cooking Time: 25 minutes

Servings: 4

Ingredients:

- 3 tablespoons extra-virgin olive oil

- 2 garlic cloves, minced

- 3 large or 4 medium zucchinis, diced

- 1/2 teaspoon freshly ground black pepper

- 1/4 teaspoon kosher or sea salt

- 1/2 cup 2% milk

- 1/4 teaspoon ground nutmeg

- 8 ounces uncooked farfalle

- 1/2 cup grated Parmesan or Romano cheese

- 1 tablespoon freshly squeezed lemon juice

Directions:

1. Heat the olive oil in a big skillet over medium heat. Add the minced garlic and stir constantly for one minute.

2. Add the diced zucchini, black pepper, and salt. Stir well, cover, and cook for 15 minutes, stirring once or twice.

3. In a small, microwave-safe bowl, warm the milk in the microwave on high for 30 seconds.

4. Stir the milk and nutmeg into the skillet and cook uncovered for another 5 minutes, stirring occasionally.

5. Meanwhile, in a large stockpot, cook the farfalle according to the package directions. Drain the pasta in a colander, saving about 2 tablespoons of pasta water.

6. Add the cooked pasta and pasta water to the skillet. Mix well, remove from heat, stir in the grated cheese and lemon juice, and serve.

Nutrition Information:

Calories: 405

Fat: 6g

Carbs: 57g

Protein: 12g

6. Pan-Fried Chili Sea Scallops

Preparation Time: 10 minutes

Cooking Time: 13-15 minutes

Servings: 4

Ingredients:

- Large sea scallops, 1/2 pound, de-tensed

- 3 tablespoons olive oil

- 1 garlic clove, finely chopped

- 1/2 teaspoon red pepper flakes

- 2 tablespoons chili sauce

- 1/4 cup tomato sauce

- 1 small shallot, minced

- 1 tablespoon minced fresh cilantro

- Salt and black pepper to taste

Directions:

1. Warm the olive oil in a skillet over medium heat. Add the scallops and cook, stirring, for 2 minutes.

2. Flip the scallops and continue to cook for 2 more minutes, without moving them, until golden browned. Set aside.

3. Add the minced shallot and garlic to the skillet and sauté for 3-5 minutes until softened. Pour in the chili sauce, tomato sauce, and red pepper flakes, and stir for 3-4 minutes.

4. Add the scallops back and warm through. Adjust the taste and top with cilantro before serving.

Nutrition Information:

Calories: 204

Fat: 4.1g

Carbs: 5g

Protein: 14g

7. Herb–Marinated Chicken Breasts

Preparation Time: 10 minutes + marinating time

Cooking Time: 10 minutes

Servings: 4

Ingredients:

- 1/2 cup fresh lemon juice

- 1/4 cup extra-virgin olive oil

- 4 cloves garlic, minced

- 2 tablespoons chopped fresh basil

- 1 tablespoon chopped fresh oregano

- 1 tablespoon chopped fresh mint

- 2 pounds chicken breast tenders

- Half a teaspoon of coarse sea salt or salt

- 1/4 teaspoon freshly ground black pepper

Directions:

1. In a small bowl, whisk together the lemon juice, olive oil, minced garlic, basil, oregano, and mint until well combined.

2. Transfer the chicken breast tenders to a wide glass baking pan or shallow basin and cover them with the herb marinade.

3. Cover, refrigerate, and allow to marinate for 1 to 2 hours. Remove from the refrigerator and season the chicken with salt and pepper.

4. Heat a large, wide skillet over medium-high heat. Using tongs, place the chicken tenders evenly in the skillet. Pour the remaining marinade over the chicken.

5. Cook for 3 to 5 minutes on each side, or until the chicken is golden, and the juices have been absorbed. Serve!

Nutrition Information:

Calories: 521

Fat: 5g

Carbs: 3g

Protein: 48g

8. Dill Salmon Salad Wraps

Preparation Time: 10 minutes

Cooking Time: 0 minutes

Servings: 6

Ingredients:

- 1 pound salmon fillet, cooked and flaked

- 1/2 cup diced carrots

- 1/2 cup diced celery

- 3 tablespoons chopped fresh dill

- 3 tablespoons diced red onion

- 2 tablespoons capers

- 1 1/2 tablespoons extra-virgin olive oil

- 1 tablespoon aged balsamic vinegar

- 1/2 teaspoon freshly ground black pepper

- 1/4 teaspoon kosher or sea salt

- 4 whole-wheat flatbread wraps

Directions:

1. In a large bowl, combine the cooked and flaked salmon with diced carrots, celery, fresh dill, red onion, capers, olive oil, balsamic vinegar, black pepper, and salt.

2. Divide the salmon salad mixture among the whole-wheat flatbreads. Fold up the bottom of each flatbread, then roll up the wraps and serve.

Nutrition Information:

Calories: 185

Fat: 8g

Carbs: 12g

Protein: 17g

9. Herbed Ricotta–Stuffed Mushrooms

Preparation Time: 10 minutes

Cooking Time: 30 minutes

Servings: 4

Ingredients:

- 6 tablespoons extra-virgin olive oil, divided

- 4 portobello mushroom caps, cleaned and gills removed

- 1 cup whole-milk ricotta cheese

- 1/3 cup chopped fresh herbs

- 2 garlic cloves, finely minced

- 1/2 teaspoon salt

- 1/4 teaspoon freshly ground black pepper

Directions:

1. Preheat the oven to 400°F and line a baking sheet with parchment or foil. Drizzle with 2 tablespoons olive oil, spreading it evenly.

2. Arrange the mushroom caps, gill-side up, on the baking sheet.

3. In a medium bowl, mix together the ricotta, herbs, 2 tablespoons olive oil, garlic, salt, and pepper.

4. Stuff each mushroom cap with one-quarter of the cheese mixture, pressing down if needed.

5. Drizzle with the remaining 2 tablespoons olive oil and bake for 30 to 35 minutes until golden brown and the mushrooms are soft.

Nutrition:

Calories: 308

Fat: 9g

Carbs: 6g

Protein: 9g

10. Hake Fillet in Herby Tomato Sauce

Preparation Time: 10 minutes

Cooking Time: 16 minutes

Servings: 4

Ingredients:

- 2 tablespoons olive oil

- 1 onion, sliced thin

- 1 fennel bulb, sliced

- 4 garlic cloves, minced

- 1 teaspoon fresh thyme, chopped

- 1 can diced tomatoes

- 1/2 cup dry white wine

- 4 skinless hake fillets

- 2 tablespoons fresh basil, chopped

- Salt and black pepper to taste

Directions:

1. Warm the olive oil in a skillet over medium heat. Sauté the onion and fennel for about 5 minutes until softened.

2. Stir in garlic and thyme and cook for about 30 seconds until fragrant. Pour in tomatoes and wine and bring to a simmer.

3. Season the hake with salt and pepper. Arrange the hake skinned side down into the tomato sauce and spoon some sauce over the top. Let it simmer.

4. Cook for 10-12 minutes until hake easily flakes with a fork. Sprinkle with basil and serve.

Nutrition:

Calories: 452

Fat: 9.9g

Carbs: 9.7g

Protein: 78g

11. Orzo-Stuffed Tomatoes

Preparation Time: 15 minutes

Cooking Time: 30 minutes

Servings: 2

Ingredients:

- 1 tablespoon olive oil

- 1 small zucchini, minced

- 1/2 medium onion, minced

- 1 garlic clove, minced

- 2/3 cup cooked orzo

- 1/2 teaspoon salt

- 2 teaspoons dried oregano

- 6 medium round tomatoes (not Roma)

Directions:

1. Preheat the oven to 350°F.

2. Heat the olive oil in a large sauté pan over medium-high heat. Add the zucchini, onion, and garlic, and sauté for 15 minutes, or until the vegetables turn golden.

3. Stir to thoroughly cook the orzo, salt, and oregano. After turning off the heat, put the pan aside.

4. Trim each tomato's top by about 1/2 inch. Using a paring knife, cut out roughly half of the tomato's flesh by cutting around its inner core.

5. Stuff the orzo mixture inside each tomato. Place the tomatoes in a baking tray and bake until they are tender, about 15 minutes.

6. They won't hold together if they are overcooked. You can serve this without roasting the tomatoes, if you'd like.

Nutrition:

Calories: 241

Fat: 8g

Carbs: 38g

Protein: 7g

12. Sautéed Lemon & Garlic Chicken

Preparation Time: 10 minutes

Cooking Time: 15 minutes

Servings: 3

Ingredients:

- Two large, thinly sliced boneless, skinless chicken breasts

- 1/4 cup extra virgin olive oil

- 3 garlic cloves, finely chopped

- 5 tablespoons fresh lemon juice

- Zest of 1 lemon

- 1/2 cup chopped fresh parsley

- 1/4 teaspoon fine sea salt

- Pinch of freshly ground black pepper

Directions:

1. In a pan large enough to hold the chicken in a single layer, heat the olive oil over medium heat.

2. Add the garlic and sauté for about 30 seconds, then add the chicken. Adjust to medium-low heat and sauté for 12 minutes until they begin to brown on the edges.

3. Add the lemon zest and lemon juice. Adjust to medium heat and let it boil.

4. Cook for about 2 minutes while using a wooden spatula to scrape any browned bits from the bottom of the pan.

5. Add the parsley, stir, then remove the pan from the heat. Transfer the chicken along with any juices to a platter. Season with the sea salt and black pepper, then serve promptly.

Nutrition:

Calories: 358

Fat: 12g

Carbs: 4g

Protein: 35g

13. Quick Shrimp Fettuccine

Preparation Time: 10 minutes

Cooking Time: 10 minutes

Servings: 4-6

Ingredients:

- 8 oz fettuccine pasta

- 1/4 cup extra-virgin olive oil

- 3 tablespoons garlic, minced

- 1 lb. large shrimp (21-25), peeled & deveined

- 1/3 cup lemon juice

- 1 tablespoon lemon zest

- 1/2 teaspoon salt

- 1/2 teaspoon freshly ground black pepper

Directions:

1. Bring a big saucepan of salted water to a boil. After adding, simmer the fettuccine for eight minutes.

2. Cook the garlic and olive oil in a large skillet over medium heat for one minute.

Toss in the shrimp and cook for 3 minutes on each side in the pot. After taking the shrimp out of the pan, set it aside.

4. Include the salt, pepper, and lemon zest and juice in the saucepan. After draining the pasta, set aside 1/2 cup of the pasta water.

5. Stir everything together in the saucepan with the lemon juice and zest after adding the pasta water.

6. Include the pasta and mix to coat it evenly. Place the spaghetti on a platter and drizzle with the cooked shrimp. Serve warm.

Nutrition:

Calories: 615

Fat: 7g

Carbs: 89g

Protein: 33g

14. Tender Pork Shoulder

Preparation Time: 10 minutes

Cooking Time: 2 hours & 10 minutes

Servings: 4

Ingredients:

- 3 tablespoons olive oil

- 2 lb. lean pork shoulder

- 1 onion, chopped

- 2 tablespoons garlic, minced

- 1 tablespoon hot paprika

- 1 tablespoon basil, chopped

- 1 cup chicken broth

- Salt & black pepper to taste

Directions:

1. Preheat the oven to 350°F.

2. Heat olive oil in a skillet and brown the pork on all sides for about 8-10 minutes; remove to a baking dish. Add onion and garlic to the skillet and sauté for 3 minutes until softened.

3. Stir in hot paprika, salt, and pepper for 1 minute and pour in chicken broth. Transfer to the baking dish, cover with aluminum foil, and bake for 90 minutes.

4. Remove the foil and continue baking for another 20 minutes until browned on top.

5. Let the pork cool for a few minutes, slice, and sprinkle with basil. Serve topped with the cooking juices.

Nutrition:

Calories: 310

Fat: 5g

Carbs: 21g

Protein: 18g

15. Grilled Eggplant and Feta Sandwiches

Preparation Time: 10 minutes

Cooking Time: 8 minutes

Servings: 2

Ingredients:

 - One medium eggplant, cut into slices that are 1/2 inch thick.

1 medium eggplant, sliced into 1/2-inch-thick slices

- 2 tablespoons olive oil

- Sea salt & freshly ground pepper, to taste

- 5 to 6 tablespoons hummus

- 4 slices whole-wheat bread, toasted

- 1 cup baby spinach leaves

- 2 oz feta cheese, softened

Directions:

1. Set a grill's temperature to medium-high on gas or charcoal. To extract the bitter juices, slice the eggplant, salt both sides, and leave it for 20 minutes.

2. Rinse the eggplant and pat dry with a paper towel. Brush the eggplant slices with olive oil and season with sea salt and freshly ground pepper.

3. Grill the eggplant for 3–4 minutes per side until lightly charred on both sides but still slightly firm in the middle.

4. Spread the hummus on the bread and top with the spinach leaves, feta, and eggplant. Top with the other slice of bread and serve warm.

Nutrition:

Calories: 516

Fat: 7g

Carbs: 59g

Protein: 14g

1. Bruschetta Chicken Burgers

Preparation Time: 15 minutes

Cooking Time: 15 minutes

Servings: 2

Ingredients:

- 1 tablespoon olive oil

- 3 tablespoons finely minced onion

- 2 garlic cloves, minced

- 1 teaspoon dried basil

- 1/4 teaspoon salt

- Three tablespoons of finely chopped sun-dried tomatoes with olive oil

- 8 oz ground chicken breast

- 3 small mozzarella balls (ciliegine), minced

Directions:

1. In a small skillet set over medium-high heat, warm the olive oil. sauté the garlic and onion for five minutes, or until they are tender. Add the basil and stir. Take out and put in a medium-sized bowl.

2. Add the salt, sun-dried tomatoes, and ground chicken and stir to combine. Mix in the mozzarella balls.

3. Divide the chicken mixture in half and form into two burgers, each about 3/4-inch thick.

4. Heat a nonstick skillet over medium-high heat and add the burgers. Cook them for 5 to 6 minutes until golden brown on the bottom. Flip and cook for 5 minutes. Serve!

Nutrition:

Calories: 301

Fat: 7g

Carbs: 6g

Protein: 32g

2. Classic Margherita Pizza

Preparation Time: 10 minutes

Cooking Time: 10 minutes

Servings: 4

Ingredients:

- All-purpose flour, for dusting

- 1 lb. premade pizza dough

- 1 (15-oz) can crushed San Marzano tomatoes, with their juices

- 2 garlic cloves

- 1 teaspoon Italian seasoning

- Pinch of sea salt, plus more as needed

- 1 1/2 teaspoons olive oil, for drizzling

- 10 slices mozzarella cheese

- 12 to 15 fresh basil leaves

Directions:

1. Preheat the oven to 475°F.

2. On a floured surface, roll out the dough to a 12-inch round and place it on a lightly floured pizza pan or baking sheet.

3. In a food processor, combine the tomatoes with their juices, garlic, Italian seasoning, and salt and process until smooth. Taste and adjust the seasoning.

4. Drizzle the olive oil over the pizza dough, then spoon the pizza sauce over the dough and spread it out evenly with the back of the spoon, leaving a 1-inch border.

5. Evenly distribute the mozzarella over the pizza. Bake for 8 to 10 minutes until the crust is cooked through and golden.

6. Remove from the oven and let it sit for 1 to 2 minutes. Top with the basil right before serving.

Nutrition:

Calories: 570

Fat: 11g

Carbs: 36g

Protein: 28g

3. Pistachio-Crusted Baked Fish

Preparation Time: 10 minutes

Cooking Time: 15-20 minutes

Servings: 4

Ingredients:

- 1/2 cup extra-virgin olive oil, divided

- 1 lb. flaky white fish (such as cod, haddock, or halibut), skin removed

- 1/2 cup shelled finely chopped pistachios

- 1/2 cup ground flaxseed

- Zest & juice of 1 lemon, divided

- 1 teaspoon ground cumin

- 1 teaspoon ground allspice

- 1/2 teaspoon salt

- 1/4 teaspoon freshly ground black pepper

Directions:

1. Preheat the oven to 400°F, and line a baking sheet with parchment paper and drizzle 2 tablespoons of olive oil over the sheet, spreading to evenly coat the bottom.

2. Cut the fish into 4 equal pieces and place on the prepared baking sheet.

3. In a small bowl, combine the pistachios, flaxseed, lemon zest, cumin, allspice, salt, and pepper. Drizzle in 1/4 cup of olive oil and stir well.

4. Divide the nut mixture evenly on top of the fish pieces. Drizzle the lemon juice and remaining 2 tbsp olive oil over the fish and bake for 15 to 20 minutes until cooked through.

5. Before serving, let it cool for five minutes.

Nutrition:

Calories: 309

Fat: 10g

Carbs: 9g

Protein: 26g

4. Bomba Chicken with Chickpeas

Preparation Time: 10 minutes

Cooking Time: 30 minutes

Servings: 4

Ingredients:

- 2 lb. boneless, skinless chicken thighs

- 2 tablespoons olive oil, divided

- 1 onion, chopped

- 3 garlic cloves, minced

- 1 cup chicken broth

- 1 tablespoon low-sodium bomba sauce or harissa

- 2 (15-oz) cans chickpeas, drained and rinsed

- 1/4 cup chopped fresh Italian parsley

- Sea salt & ground black pepper to taste

Directions:

1. Make sure to liberally season the chicken thighs with salt & pepper.

2. Heat one tablespoon of olive oil in a big skillet over medium-high heat. Add the chicken and heat for 2 to 3 minutes on each side, or until browned.

3. Place the chicken on a platter and keep it there.

4. Heat the final tablespoon of olive oil in the same skillet. When the onion and garlic start to soften, sauté them for four to five minutes.

5. Return the chicken to the skillet, then add the broth and bomba sauce. Let it boil, adjust to low heat, cover, and simmer for 15 minutes, or until the chicken is cooked through.

6. Add the chickpeas and simmer for 5 minutes more. Garnish with the parsley and serve.

Nutrition:

Calories: 552

Fat: 9g

Carbs: 37g

Protein: 56g

5. Ratatouille

Preparation Time: 10 minutes

Cooking Time: 20 minutes

Servings: 4

Ingredients:

- 4 tablespoons extra-virgin olive oil, divided

- 1 cup diced zucchini

- 2 cups diced eggplant

- 1 cup diced onion

- 1 cup chopped green bell pepper

- 1 can no-salt-added diced tomatoes

- 1/2 teaspoon garlic powder

- 1 teaspoon ground thyme

- Salt & freshly ground black pepper, to taste

Directions:

1. Heat 2 tablespoons of olive oil in a large saucepan over medium heat until it shimmers.

2. Add the zucchini and eggplant and sauté for 10 minutes, stirring occasionally. Add the remaining olive oil if needed.

3. Stir in the onion and bell pepper and sauté for 5 minutes until softened.

4. Add the diced tomatoes with their juice, garlic powder, and thyme and stir to combine.

5. Continue cooking for 15 minutes until the vegetables are cooked through, stirring occasionally. Sprinkle with salt and black pepper. Serve!

Nutrition:

Calories: 189

Fat: 3.7g

Carbs: 14.8g

Protein: 3.1g

6. Pork Chops in Tomato Olive Sauce

Preparation Time: 10 minutes

Cooking Time: 10 minutes

Servings: 4

Ingredients:

- 2 tablespoons olive oil

- 4 lean pork loin chops, boneless

- 6 tomatoes, crushed

- 3 tablespoons basil, chopped

- 10 black olives, halved

- 1 yellow onion, chopped

- 1 garlic clove, minced

Directions:

1. Warm the olive oil in a skillet over medium heat and brown pork chops for 6 minutes on all sides. Share into plates.

2. In the same skillet, stir tomatoes, basil, olives, onion, and garlic and simmer for 4 minutes. Drizzle tomato sauce over.

Nutrition:

Calories: 340

Fat: 8g

Carbs: 13g

Protein: 35g

7. Olive & Escarole Salmon

Preparation Time: 10 minutes

Cooking Time: 15 minutes

Servings: 4

Ingredients:

- 3 tablespoons olive oil

- 1 head escarole, torn

- 4 salmon fillets, boneless

- Juice of 1 lime

- Salt & black pepper to taste

- 1/4 cup fish stock

- 1/4 cup green olives, pitted & chopped

- 1/4 cup fresh chives, chopped

Directions:

1. Heat half of the olive oil in a skillet over medium heat and sauté escarole, lime juice, salt, pepper, fish stock, and olives for 6 minutes. Share into plates.

2. Warm the remaining oil in the same skillet. Sprinkle salmon with salt and pepper and fry for 8 minutes on both sides until golden brown.

3. Transfer to the escarole plates and serve warm topped with chives.

Nutrition:

Calories: 280

Fat: 5g

Carbs: 25g

Protein: 19g

8. Moroccan Lamb Wrap with Harissa

Preparation Time: 20 minutes + marinating time

Cooking Time: 15 minutes

Servings: 4

Ingredients:

- 1 clove garlic, minced

- 2 teaspoons ground cumin

- 2 teaspoons chopped fresh thyme

- 1/4 cup olive oil, divided

- 1 lean lamb leg steak, about 12 oz

- 4 (8-inch) pocketless pita rounds or naan, preferably whole-wheat

- 1 medium eggplant, sliced 1/2-inch thick

- 1 medium zucchini, sliced lengthwise into 4 slices

- 1 bell pepper (any color), roasted & skinned

- 6 to 8 Kalamata olives, sliced

- Juice of 1 lemon

- 2 to 4 tablespoons harissa

- 2 cups arugula

Directions:

1. Combine the garlic, thyme, cumin, and 1 tablespoon of olive oil in a large bowl. The lamb should be added, coated, covered, chilled, and marinated for at least an hour.

2. Preheat the oven to 400°F, and heat a grill or grill pan to high heat.

3. Remove the lamb from the marinade and grill for about 4 minutes per side, until medium-rare.

4. Transfer to a plate and let it rest for about 10 minutes before slicing thinly across the grain.

5. Wrap the bread rounds in aluminum foil and heat in the oven for about 10 minutes.

6. Meanwhile, brush the eggplant and zucchini slices with the remaining olive oil and grill until tender, about 3 minutes. Dice them and the bell pepper.

7. Toss in a large bowl with the olives and lemon juice.

8. Spread some of the harissa onto each warm flatbread round and top each evenly with roasted vegetables, a few slices of lamb, and a handful of the arugula.

9. Roll up the wraps, cut each in half crosswise, and serve immediately.

Nutrition:

Calories: 553

Fat: 4g

Carbs: 53g

Protein: 33g

9. Baked Falafel Sliders

Preparation Time: 10 minutes

Cooking Time: 30 minutes

Servings: 6 sliders

Ingredients:

- Olive oil cooking spray

- 1 (15-oz) can no-salt-added or low-sodium chickpeas, drained & rinsed

- 1 onion, roughly chopped

- 2 garlic cloves, peeled

- 2 tablespoons fresh parsley, chopped

- 2 tablespoons whole-wheat flour

- 1/2 teaspoon ground coriander

- 1/2 teaspoon ground cumin

- 1/2 teaspoon baking powder

- 1/2 teaspoon kosher salt

- 1/4 teaspoon freshly ground black pepper

Directions:

1. Preheat the oven to 350ºF, and line a baking sheet with parchment paper or foil and lightly spray with olive oil cooking spray.

2. In a food processor, add the chickpeas, onion, garlic, parsley, flour, coriander, cumin, baking powder, salt, and black pepper.

3. Process until smooth, stopping to scrape down the sides of the bowl. Make 6 slider patties, each with a heaping 1/4 cup of mixture, and arrange on the prepared baking sheet.

4. Bake for 30 minutes, turning over halfway through. Serve!

Nutrition:

Calories: 90

Fat: 1g

Carbs: 17g

Protein: 4g

10. Spicy Tomato and Caper Squid Stew

Preparation time: 15 minutes

Cooking time: 47-50 minutes

Servings: 4

Ingredients:

- 1 can whole peeled tomatoes, diced

- 1/4 cup olive oil

- 1 onion, chopped

- 1 celery rib, sliced

- 3 garlic cloves, minced

- 1/4 tsp red pepper flakes

- 1 red chili, minced

- 1/2 cup dry white wine

- 2 lb. squid, sliced into rings

- Salt & black pepper to taste

- 1/3 cup green olives, chopped

- 1 tbsp capers

- 2 tbsp fresh parsley, chopped

Directions:

1. In a pot over medium heat, preheat the olive oil. For about five minutes, sauté the onion, garlic, red chile, and celery until they are tender. Add the pepper flakes and stir; simmer for 30 seconds or so.

2. Cook for 1 minute, or until almost evaporated, after stirring in the wine and scraping off any browned parts. Season with salt and pepper and add one cup of water.

3. Stir the squid into the pot. Adjust to low heat, cover, and simmer for 15 minutes until the squid has released its liquid.

4. Pour in tomatoes, olives, and capers, and cook for 30-35 minutes until squid is very tender. Top with parsley. Serve and enjoy!

Nutrition:

Calories: 334

Fat: 12g

Carbs: 30g

Protein: 28g

11. Harissa Yogurt Chicken Thighs

Preparation time: 10 minutes + marinating time

Cooking time: 25 minutes

Servings: 4

Ingredients:

- 1/2 cup low-fat plain yogurt

- 2 tbsp harissa

- 1 tbsp lemon juice

- 1/2 tsp kosher salt

- 1/4 tsp freshly ground black pepper

- 1 1/2 lb. boneless, skinless chicken thighs

Directions:

1. In a bowl, combine the yogurt, harissa, lemon juice, salt, and black pepper. Add the chicken and mix together. Marinate for at least 15 minutes, and up to 4 hours in the refrigerator.

2. Preheat the oven to 425°F, and line a baking sheet with parchment paper or foil. Remove the chicken thighs from the marinade and arrange in one layer on the baking sheet.

3. Roast for 20 minutes, turning the chicken over halfway. Adjust to a broil. Broil the chicken for 2 to 3 minutes until golden brown in spots.

Nutrition:

Calories: 190

Fat: 10g

Carbs: 1g

Protein: 24g

12. Baked Asparagus Caprese Pasta

Preparation time: 10 minutes

Cooking time: 20 minutes

Servings: 6

Ingredients:

- 8 oz uncooked small pasta

- 1½ lb. fresh asparagus, ends trimmed & stalks chopped into 1-inch pieces

- 1 ½ cup grape tomatoes, halved

- 2 tbsp extra-virgin olive oil

- ¼ tsp freshly ground black pepper

- ¼ tsp kosher or sea salt

- 2 cups fresh mozzarella, drained & cut into bite-size pieces

- 1/3 cup torn fresh basil leaves

- 2 tbsp balsamic vinegar

Directions:

1. Preheat the oven to 400°F.

2. In a large stockpot, cook the pasta according to the package directions. Drain, reserving about ¼ cup of the pasta water.

3. In a large bowl, toss the asparagus, tomatoes, oil, pepper, and salt together. Spread the mixture onto a large, rimmed baking sheet and bake for 15 minutes, stirring twice as it cooks.

4. Remove the vegetables from the oven and add the cooked pasta to the baking sheet.

5. Mix with a few tablespoons of pasta water to help the sauce become smoother and the saucy vegetables stick to the pasta.

6. Gently mix in the mozzarella and basil. Drizzle with the balsamic vinegar. Serve from the baking sheet or pour the pasta into a large bowl.

Nutrition:

Calories: 317

Fat: 12g

Carbs: 38g

Protein: 16g

13. Lemon Trout with Roasted Beets

Preparation time: 15 minutes

Cooking time: 36 minutes

Servings: 4

Ingredients:

- 1 lb. medium beets, peeled & sliced

- 3 tbsp olive oil

- 4 trout fillets, boneless

- Salt & black pepper to taste

- 1 tbsp rosemary, chopped

- 2 spring onions, chopped

- 2 tbsp lemon juice

- ½ cup vegetable stock

Directions:

1. Preheat the oven to 390°F and line a baking sheet with parchment paper.

2. Arrange the beets on the sheet, season with salt and pepper, and drizzle with some olive oil. Roast for 20 minutes.

3. Warm the remaining oil in a skillet over medium heat. Cook trout fillets for 8 minutes on all sides; reserve. Add spring onions to the skillet and sauté for 2 minutes.

4. Stir in lemon juice and stock and cook for 5-6 minutes until the sauce thickens. Remove the beets to a plate and top with trout fillets. Pour the sauce all over and sprinkle with rosemary.

Nutrition:

Calories: 240

Fat: 6g

Carbs: 22g

Protein: 18g

14. Date Lamb Tagine

Preparation time: 10 minutes

Cooking time: 30 minutes

Servings: 4

Ingredients:

- 2 tbsp olive oil

- 1 tbsp chopped dates

- 1 lb. lean lamb, cubed

- 1 garlic clove, minced

- 1 onion, grated

- 2 tbsp orange juice

- Salt & black pepper to taste

- 1 cup vegetable stock

Directions:

1. Warm the olive oil in a skillet over medium heat and cook onion and garlic for 5 minutes. Add lamb and cook for another 5 minutes.

2. Stir in dates, orange juice, salt, pepper, and stock and bring to a boil; cook for 20 minutes. Serve.

Nutrition:

Calories: 298

Fat: 14g

Carbs: 19g

Protein: 17g

15. Fennel Poached Cod with Tomatoes

Preparation time: 10 minutes

Cooking time: 20 minutes

Servings: 4

Ingredients:

- 1 tbsp olive oil

- 1 cup thinly sliced fennel

- ½ cup thinly sliced onion

- 1 tbsp minced garlic

- 1 can diced tomatoes

- 2 cups chicken broth

- ½ cup white wine

- Juice & zest of 1 orange

- 1 pinch red pepper flakes

- 1 bay leaf

- 1 lb. cod fillet

Directions:

1. In a big skillet, heat the olive oil. Add the onion and fennel and simmer, stirring occasionally, until the vegetables are transparent, about 6 minutes. Another minute is added when you add the garlic.

2. Add the tomatoes, chicken broth, wine, orange juice and zest, red pepper flakes, and bay leaf, and simmer for 5 minutes to meld the flavors.

3. Carefully add the cod in a single layer, cover, and simmer for 6 to 7 minutes. Transfer fish to a serving dish, ladle the remaining sauce over the fish, and serve.

Nutrition:

Calories: 336

Fat: 12.5g

Carbs: 11.0g

Protein: 45.1g

1. Zesty Feta and Olive Blend

Preparation time: 10 minutes

Cooking time: 0 minutes

Servings: 8

Ingredients:

- 1 (1 lb.) block of feta cheese, cut into ½-inch squares

- 3 cups mixed olives, drained from brine; pitted preferred

- ¼ cup extra-virgin olive oil

- 3 tbsp lemon juice

- 1 tsp grated lemon zest

- 1 tsp dried oregano

- Pita bread, for serving

Directions:

1. Place the feta cheese into a large bowl. Add the olives to the feta and set aside.

2. In a small bowl, whisk the olive oil, lemon juice, lemon zest, and oregano.

3. Pour the dressing over the feta cheese and olives and gently toss together to evenly coat everything. Serve with pita bread.

Nutrition: Calories: 269; Fat: 4g; Carbs: 6g; Protein: 9g

2. Garlic-infused Broccoli Rabe with Artichokes

Prep time: 10 minutes

Cooking time: 10 minutes

Servings: 4

Ingredients:

- 2 lb. fresh broccoli rabe

- ½ cup extra-virgin olive oil, divided

- 3 garlic cloves, finely minced

- 1 tsp salt

- 1 tsp red pepper flakes

- 1 (13¾-oz) can artichoke hearts, drained and quartered

- 1 tbsp water

- 2 tbsp red wine vinegar

- Freshly ground black pepper to taste

Directions:

1. Trim away any thick lower stems and yellow leaves from the broccoli rabe and discard. Cut into individual florets with a couple of inches of thin stem attached.

2. In a large skillet, heat ¼ cup olive oil over medium-high heat. Add the trimmed broccoli, garlic, salt, and red pepper flakes and sauté for 5 minutes, until the broccoli begins to soften.

3. Add the artichoke hearts and sauté for another 2 minutes. Add the water and reduce the heat to low. Cover and simmer for 3 to 5 minutes until the broccoli stems are tender.

4. In a small bowl, whisk together the remaining ¼ cup olive oil and the vinegar. Drizzle over the broccoli and artichokes. Season with ground black pepper, if desired.

Nutrition: Calories: 341; Fat: 8g; Carbs: 18g; Protein: 11g

3. Greens Braised with Olives and Walnuts

Preparation time: 10 minutes

Cooking time: 20 minutes

Servings: 4

Ingredients:

- 8 cups fresh greens, chopped into bite-size pieces

 - Two to four finely minced garlic cloves

- ½ cup roughly chopped pitted green or black olives

- ½ cup roughly chopped shelled walnuts

- ¼ cup extra-virgin olive oil

- 2 tbsp red wine vinegar

- 1 to 2 tsp freshly chopped herbs

Directions:

1. Place the greens in a large rimmed skillet or pot. Turn the heat to high and add the minced garlic and enough water to just cover the greens.

2. Bring to a boil, then adjust to low heat and simmer until the greens are wilted and tender, and most of the liquid has evaporated, adding more water if the greens start to burn.

3. Once cooked, remove from the heat and add the chopped olives and walnuts.

4. In a small bowl, whisk together olive oil, vinegar, and herbs. Drizzle over the cooked greens and toss to coat. Serve warm.

Nutrition: Calories: 254; Fat: 5g; Carbs: 6g; Protein: 4g

4. Roasted Honey Acorn Squash

Preparation time: 10 minutes

Cooking time: 30 minutes

Servings: 4

Ingredients:

- 1 acorn squash, cut into wedges

- 2 tbsp olive oil

- 2 tbsp honey

- 2 tbsp rosemary, chopped

- 2 tbsp walnuts, chopped

Directions:

1. Preheat the oven to 400°F.

2. In a bowl, mix the honey, rosemary, and olive oil. Lay the squash wedges on a baking sheet and drizzle with the honey mixture.

3. Bake for 30 minutes until the squash is tender and slightly caramelized, turning each slice over halfway through. Serve cooled, sprinkled with walnuts.

Nutrition: Calories: 136; Fat: 6g; Carbs: 20g; Protein: 0.9g

5. Oven-Baked Beet and Leek with Dilly Yogurt

Preparation time: 10 minutes

Cooking time: 30 minutes

Servings: 4

Ingredients:

- 5 tbsp olive oil

- ½ lb. leeks, thickly sliced

- 1 lb. red beets, sliced

- 1 cup plain low-fat yogurt

- 2 garlic cloves, finely minced

- ¼ tsp ground cumin

- ¼ tsp dried parsley

- ¼ cup chopped parsley

- 1 tsp dill

- Salt & black pepper to taste

Directions:

1. Preheat the oven to 390°F. Arrange the beets and leeks on a greased roasting dish. Sprinkle with olive oil, cumin, dried parsley, black pepper, and salt.

2. Bake in the oven for 25-30 minutes. Transfer to a serving platter.

3. In a bowl, stir together yogurt, dill, garlic, and the remaining olive oil. Whisk to combine. Drizzle the veggies with the yogurt sauce and top with fresh parsley to serve.

Nutrition: Calories: 281; Fat: 8.7g; Carbs: 24g; Protein: 6g

6. Wok-Style Kale with Mushrooms

Preparation time: 10 minutes

Cooking time: 9 minutes

Servings: 4

Ingredients:

- 1 cup cremini mushrooms, sliced

- 4 tbsp olive oil

- 1 small red onion, chopped

- 2 cloves garlic, thinly sliced

- 1 ½ lb. curly kale

- 2 tomatoes, chopped

- 1 tsp dried oregano

- 1 tsp dried basil

- ½ tsp dried rosemary

- ½ tsp dried thyme

- Salt & black pepper to taste

Directions:

1. In a saucepan over medium heat, warm the olive oil. Add the onion and garlic and sauté until softened, about 3 minutes.

2. Add the mushrooms, kale, and tomatoes, stirring to promote even cooking. Turn the heat to a simmer, add the spices, and cook for 5-6 minutes until the kale wilts.

Nutrition: Calories: 221; Fat: 6g; Carbs: 19g; Protein: 9g

7. Dandelion Greens Sautéed with Sweet Onion

Preparation time: 10 minutes

Cooking time: 10 minutes

Servings: 4

Ingredients:

- 1 tbsp extra-virgin olive oil

- 2 garlic cloves, minced

- 1 Vidalia onion, thinly sliced

- ½ cup low-sodium vegetable broth

- 2 bunches dandelion greens, roughly chopped

- Freshly ground black pepper, to taste

Directions:

1. In a big skillet over low heat, warm the olive oil.

2. Add the garlic and onion, and cook for 2 to 3 minutes, stirring occasionally, until the onion is translucent.

3. Fold in the vegetable broth and dandelion greens, and cook for 5 to 7 minutes until wilted, stirring frequently.

4. Sprinkle with black pepper and serve on a plate while warm.

Nutrition: Calories: 81; Fat: 3.9g; Carbs: 10.8g; Protein: 3.2g

8. Zesty Zucchini Cubes with Mint

Preparation time: 10 minutes

Cooking time: 10 minutes

Servings: 4

Ingredients:

- 3 large green zucchinis, cut into ½-inch cubes

- 3 tbsp extra-virgin olive oil

- 1 large onion, chopped

- 3 cloves garlic, minced

- 1 tsp salt

- 1 tsp dried mint

Directions:

1. In a big skillet over medium heat, warm the olive oil. Add the onion and garlic, and sauté, stirring frequently, for 3 minutes, or until the ingredients soften.

2. Stir in the zucchini cubes and salt, and cook for 5 minutes, until the zucchini is browned and tender.

3. Add the mint to the skillet, toss to combine, and continue cooking for 2 minutes. Serve warm.

Nutrition: Calories: 146; Fat: 10.6g; Carbs: 11.8g; Protein: 4.2g

9. Herbed Marinated Mushrooms and Olives

Preparation time: 10 minutes + marinating time

Cooking time: 0 minutes

Servings: 8

Ingredients:

- 1 lb. white button mushrooms

- 1 lb. mixed, high-quality olives

- 2 tbsp fresh thyme leaves

- 1 tbsp white wine vinegar

- ½ tbsp crushed fennel seeds

- Pinch of chili flakes

- Olive oil, to cover

- Sea salt & freshly ground pepper, to taste

Directions:

1. Combine all ingredients in a glass jar or other airtight container. Cover with olive oil and season with sea salt and freshly ground pepper.

2. Shake to distribute the ingredients. Allow to marinate for at least 1 hour. Serve at room temperature.

Nutrition: Calories: 61; Fat: 4g; Carbs: 5g; Protein: 2g

10. Parmesan Roasted Cauliflower and Tomatoes

Preparation time: 5 minutes

Cooking time: 25 minutes

Servings: 4

Ingredients:

- 4 cups cauliflower, cut into 1-inch pieces

- 6 tbsp extra-virgin olive oil, divided

- 1 tsp salt, divided

- 4 cups cherry tomatoes

- ½ tsp freshly ground black pepper

- ½ cup grated Parmesan cheese

Directions:

1. Preheat the oven to 425°F.

2. In a large bowl, toss cauliflower with 3 tablespoons of olive oil and ½ teaspoon of salt. Spread the cauliflower on a baking sheet in an even layer.

3. Transfer the tomatoes to another bowl and toss them with the remaining 3 tablespoons olive oil and ½ teaspoon salt. Arrange the tomatoes onto each individual baking sheet.

4. Roast both sheets in the oven for 17 to 20 minutes until the cauliflower is lightly browned, and the tomatoes are plump.

5. Spoon the roasted cauliflower into a serving dish, top with tomatoes, black pepper, and Parmesan cheese. Serve warm.

Nutrition: Calories: 294; Fat: 6g; Carbs: 13g; Protein: 9g

1. Bucatini in Puttanesca Style

Preparation time: 10 minutes

Cooking time: 25 minutes

Servings: 4

Ingredients:

- 1 tbsp capers, rinsed

- 1 tsp coarsely chopped fresh oregano

- 1 tsp finely chopped garlic

- 1/8 tsp salt

- 12-oz bucatini pasta, cooked & drained

- 2 cups coarsely chopped canned no-salt-added whole peeled tomatoes with their juice

- Split 3 tablespoons extra virgin olive oil.

- 4 anchovy fillets, chopped

- 8 black Kalamata olives, pitted & sliced into slivers

Directions:

1. Heat 2 tbsp oil in a large nonstick saucepan over medium heat.

2. Sauté the anchovies until they start to disintegrate. Add garlic and sauté for 15 seconds.

3. Add tomatoes, sauté for 15 to 20 minutes or until no longer watery; season with 1/8 tsp salt.

4. Add oregano, capers, and olives. Add pasta, sautéing until heated through. Drizzle leftover olive oil over pasta before serving and enjoy.

Nutrition: Calories: 207; Fat: 12g; Carbs: 31g; Protein: 5.1g

2. White Bean Lettuce Wraps

Preparation time: 10 minutes

Cooking time: 9 minutes

Servings: 4

Ingredients:

- 1 tbsp extra-virgin olive oil

- ½ cup diced red onion

- ¾ cup chopped fresh tomatoes

- ¼ tsp freshly ground black pepper

- 1 (15-oz) can cannellini or great northern beans, drained & rinsed

- ¼ cup finely chopped fresh curly parsley

- ½ cup low-sodium lemony garlic hummus

- 8 romaine lettuce leaves

Directions:

1. Heat the oil in a big skillet over medium heat. Add the onion and simmer, stirring periodically, for two to three minutes.

2. Add the tomatoes and pepper and cook for 3 more minutes, stirring occasionally.

3. Add the beans and cook for 3 more minutes, stirring occasionally. Remove from the heat and mix in the parsley.

4. Spread 1 tbsp of hummus over each lettuce leaf. Evenly spread the warm bean mixture down the center of each leaf.

5. Fold one side of the lettuce leaf over the filling lengthwise, then fold over the other side to make a wrap and serve.

Nutrition: Calories: 188; Fat: 5g; Carbs: 28g; Protein: 10g

3. Mango Infused Chili Black Beans

Preparation time: 10 minutes

Cooking time: 10 minutes

Servings: 4

Ingredients:

- 2 tbsp coconut oil

- 1 onion, chopped

- 2 (15-oz) cans black beans, drained & rinsed

- 1 tbsp chili powder

- 1 tsp sea salt

- ¼ tsp freshly ground black pepper

- 1 cup water

- 2 ripe mangoes, thinly sliced

- ¼ cup chopped fresh cilantro, divided

- ¼ cup sliced scallions, divided

Directions:

1. In a pot over high heat, melt the coconut oil. Add the chopped onion and cook until transparent, about 5 minutes.

2. Fill the pot with the black beans. Add salt, ground black pepper, and chili powder. Add water to the mixture. Mix thoroughly by stirring.

3. Bring to a boil. Reduce the heat to low, then simmer for 5 minutes or until the beans are tender.

4. Turn off the heat and gently fold in the mango slices. Garnish with scallions and cilantro before serving.

Nutrition: Calories: 277; Fat: 9g; Carbs: 45g; Protein: 4g

4. Fava Bean and Garbanzo Fūl

Preparation time: 10 minutes

Cooking time: 10 minutes

Servings: 6

Ingredients:

- 1 (16-oz) can garbanzo beans, rinsed & drained

- 1 (15- oz) can fava beans, rinsed & drained

- 3 cups water

- ½ cup lemon juice

- 3 cloves garlic, peeled & minced

- 1 tsp salt

- 3 tbsp extra-virgin olive oil

Directions:

1. In a 3-quart pot over medium heat, cook the garbanzo beans, fava beans, and water for 10 minutes.

2. Reserving 1 cup of the liquid from the cooked beans, drain the beans and place them in a container.

3. Mix the reserved liquid, lemon juice, minced garlic, and salt together; add to the beans in the container. Mash about half the beans with a potato masher.

4. After mashing half the beans, stir the mixture once more to ensure even mixing.

5. Drizzle the olive oil over the top. Serve with pita bread warm or cold.

Nutrition: Calories: 199; Fat: 9g; Carbs: 25g; Protein: 10g

5. White Cannellini Bean Stew

Preparation time: 10 minutes

Cooking time: 30 minutes

Servings: 4-6

Ingredients:

- 3 tbsp extra-virgin olive oil

- 1 large onion, chopped

- 1 (15-oz) can diced tomatoes

- 2 (15-oz) cans white cannellini beans

- 1 cup carrots, chopped

- 4 cups vegetable broth

- 1 tsp salt

- 1 (1 lb.) bag baby spinach, washed

Directions:

1. Cook the onion and olive oil in a big pot over medium heat for five minutes. Add the salt, broth, carrots, beans, and tomatoes. Cook for 20 minutes while stirring.

2. Add the spinach, a handful at a time, and cook for 5 minutes until the spinach has wilted. Serve warm.

Nutrition: Calories: 356; Fat: 12g; Carbs: 47g; Protein: 15g.

6. Halloumi and Green Bean Salad

Preparation time: 15 minutes

Cooking time: 6 minutes

Servings: 2

Ingredients:

For the Dressing:

- ¼ cup plain kefir or buttermilk

- 1 tbsp olive oil

- 2 tsp freshly squeezed lemon juice

- ¼ tsp onion powder

- ¼ tsp garlic powder

- pinch of salt & freshly ground black pepper

For the Salad:

- ½ lb. very fresh green beans, trimmed

- 2 oz Halloumi cheese, sliced into 2 (½-inch-thick) slices

- ½ cup cherry or grape tomatoes, halved

- ¼ cup of sweet onion, thinly sliced

Directions:

1. Combine the kefir or buttermilk, olive oil, lemon juice, onion powder, garlic powder, salt, and pepper in a small container and whisk well. Set the dressing aside.

2. Fill a medium-size pot with about 1 inch of water and add the green beans. Cover and steam them for about 3 to 4 minutes, or just until beans are tender. Do not overcook.

3. Drain the beans, rinse them immediately with cold water, and set them aside to cool.

4. Heat a nonstick skillet over medium-high heat and place the slices of Halloumi into the hot pan. After about 2 minutes, check to see if the cheese is golden on the bottom.

5. If it is, flip the slices and cook for another minute or until the second side is golden. Remove cheese and cut each piece into cubes (about 1-inch square).

6. Place the green beans, halloumi, tomatoes, and sliced onion in a large container and toss to combine.

7. Drizzle dressing over the salad and toss well to combine. Serve.

Nutrition: Calories: 273; Fat: 8g; Carbs: 16g; Protein: 15g.

7. Tuscan-Style Baked Beans

Preparation time: 10 minutes

Cooking time: 15 minutes

Servings: 6

Ingredients:

- 2 tsp extra-virgin olive oil

- ½ cup minced onion

- 1 (12-oz) can low-sodium tomato paste

- ¼ cup red wine vinegar

- 2 tbsp honey

- ¼ tsp ground cinnamon

- ½ cup water

- 2 (15-oz) cans cannellini or great northern beans, undrained

Directions:

1. Heat the oil in a medium saucepan over medium heat. Stir often for 5 minutes after adding the onion.

2. Add the tomato paste, vinegar, honey, cinnamon, and water and stir well. Lower the heat to low.

3. Drain and rinse one can of beans in a colander and add to the saucepan. Pour the entire second can of beans (including the liquid) into the casserole.

4. Cook for 10 minutes, stirring occasionally, and serve.

Nutrition: Calories: 290; Fat: 2g; Carbs: 53g; Protein: 15g

8. Pinto Bean Salad

Preparation time: 10 minutes

Cooking time: 3 minutes

Servings: 4-6

Ingredients:

- ¼ cup extra-virgin olive oil, divided

- - Three peeled and gently smashed garlic cloves

- 2 (15-oz) cans pinto beans, rinsed

- 2 cups + 1 tbsp water

- salt & pepper, to taste

- ¼ cup tahini

- 3 tbsp lemon juice

- 1 tbsp ground dried Aleppo pepper, + extra for serving

- 8 oz cherry tomatoes, halved

- ¼ red onion, sliced thinly

- ½ cup fresh parsley leaves

- 2 hard-cooked large eggs, quartered

- 1 tbsp toasted sesame seeds

Directions:

1. Add 1 tablespoon olive oil and the garlic to a medium saucepan over medium heat. Cook for about 3 minutes, stirring constantly, or until garlic turns golden brown but not brown.

2. Include the beans and bring to a boil, adding 2 cups of water and 1 tablespoon of salt. After removing from the heat, cover and leave for 20 minutes. Remove the garlic and drain the beans.

3. In a large bowl, whisk the remaining 3 tablespoons oil, tahini, lemon juice, Aleppo, the remaining 1 tablespoon water, and ¼ teaspoon salt. Stir in the beans, tomatoes, onion, and parsley.

4. Season with salt and pepper to taste. Transfer to a serving dish and top with the eggs. Sprinkle with the extra sesame and Aleppo seeds before serving.

Nutrition: Calories: 402; Fat: 8g; Carbs: 44g; Protein: 16g

9. Yogurt and Chickpea Delight

Preparation time: 10 minutes

Cooking time: 10 minutes

Servings: 4

Ingredients:

- 4 cups plain low-fat yogurt

- 3 cloves garlic, minced

- 1 tsp salt

- - Two 16-oz cans of washed and drained garbanzo beans

- 2 cups water

- 4 cups pita chips

- 5 tbsp unsalted butter (optional)

Directions:

1. In a large bowl, whisk together the yogurt, minced garlic, and salt. Set aside.

2. Place the garbanzo beans and water in a medium pot, bring to a boil, and let the beans boil for about 5 minutes.

3. Pour the garbanzo beans and the cooking liquid into a large casserole dish. Top the beans with pita chips. Pour the yogurt sauce over the pita chip layer.

4. In a small saucepan, melt and brown the butter (if desired) for about 3 minutes. Drizzle the brown butter over the yogurt sauce.

Nutrition: Calories: 272; Fat: 6g; Carbs: 33g; Protein: 39g

10. Golden Organic Chickpeas

Preparation time: 10 minutes

Cooking time: 30 minutes

Servings: 4

Ingredients:

- 2 (15-oz) cans organic chickpeas, drained & rinsed

- 3 tbsp extra-virgin olive oil

- 2 tsp smoked paprika

- 2 tsp turmeric

- ½ tsp dried oregano

- ½ tsp salt

- ¼ tsp ground ginger

- 1/8 tsp ground white pepper (optional)

Directions:

1. Preheat the oven to 400ºF, line a baking sheet with parchment paper, and set aside.

2. Pat the chickpeas completely dry, lay them on a baking sheet, roll them around with paper towels, and let them air-dry for at least 3 hours, or overnight.

3. In a medium bowl, combine the olive oil, smoked paprika, turmeric, oregano, salt, ginger, and white pepper (if using).

4. Include the desiccated chickpeas in the dish and mix thoroughly.

5. Spread the chickpeas on the prepared baking sheet and bake for 30 minutes or until golden brown.

6. After 15 minutes, stir the chickpeas on the baking sheet to prevent burning.

7. Check every 10 minutes to ensure the chickpeas don't crisp up too quickly. Let them cool and serve.

Nutrition: Calories: 308; Fat: 12g; Carbs: 40g; Protein: 11g

1. Hummus-Cucumber Delight

Preparation time: 10 minutes

Cooking time: 0 minutes

Servings: 2

Ingredients:

- 4 slices whole-grain bread

- ¼ cup hummus

- 1 large cucumber, thinly sliced

- 4 whole basil leaves

Directions:

1. Spread the hummus on 2 slices of bread, and layer the cucumbers onto it.

2. Top with the basil leaves and close the sandwiches. Press down lightly and serve immediately.

Nutrition: Calories: 209; Fat: 5g; Carbs: 32g; Protein: 9g

2. Feta and Artichoke Medley

Preparation time: 10 minutes

Cooking time: 0 minutes

Servings: 1½ cups

Ingredients:

- 4 oz low-fat feta, cut into ½-inch cubes

- 4 oz drained artichoke hearts, quartered lengthwise

- 1/3 cup extra-virgin olive oil

- Zest & juice of 1 lemon

- 2 tbsp roughly chopped fresh rosemary

- 2 tbsp roughly chopped fresh parsley

- ½ tsp black peppercorns

Directions:

1. In a glass bowl or large glass jar, combine the feta and artichoke hearts.

2. Add the olive oil, lemon zest and juice, rosemary, parsley, and peppercorns, and toss gently to coat, being sure not to crumble the feta.

3. Cover and refrigerate for at least 4 hours, or up to 4 days. Pull out of the refrigerator 30 minutes before serving.

Nutrition: Calories: 108; Fat: 9g; Carbs: 4g; Protein: 3g

3. Maple-Spiced Nut Medley

Preparation time: 10 minutes

Cooking time: 10 minutes

Servings: 2 cups

Ingredients:

- 2 cups raw walnuts or pecans (or a mix of nuts)

- 1 tsp extra-virgin olive oil

- 1 tsp ground sumac

- ½ tsp pure maple syrup

- ¼ tsp kosher salt

- ¼ tsp ground ginger

- 2 to 4 rosemary sprigs

Directions:

1. Preheat the oven to 350°F, and line a baking sheet with parchment paper or foil.

2. Place the nuts, ginger, maple syrup, sumac, olive oil, and salt in a big bowl and stir to incorporate. Arrange on the prepared baking sheet in a single layer. Incorporate the rosemary.

3. Roast until fragrant and golden, 8 to 10 minutes. Take the leaves off of the rosemary stalks and transfer them to a serving basin. Before serving, add the nuts and stir to incorporate.

Nutrition: Calories: 175; Fat: 8g; Carbs: 4g; Protein: 3g

4. Arugula Pesto Dip

Preparation time: 10 minutes

Cooking time: 0 minutes

Servings: 4

Ingredients:

- 1 cup arugula, chopped

- 3 tbsp basil pesto

- 1 cup cream cheese, softened

- Salt & black pepper to taste

- 1 cup heavy cream

- 1 tbsp chives, chopped

Directions:

1. Combine arugula, basil pesto, salt, pepper, and heavy cream in a blender and pulse until smooth.

2. Pour into a bowl and incorporate cream cheese. Garnish with chives and serve.

Nutrition: Calories: 240; Fat: 15g; Carbs: 7g; Protein: 6g

5. Citrus-Spiced Nut Mix

Preparation time: 10 minutes

Cooking time: 20 minutes

Servings: 10-12

Ingredients:

- Nonstick cooking spray

- Zest & juice of 1 lemon

- 2 tbsp honey

- 2 tsp Berbere or baharat spice blend

- 1 tsp Aleppo pepper

- 1½ cups cashews

- 1½ cups dry-roasted peanuts

Directions:

1. Preheat the oven to 375°F and line a baking sheet with parchment paper, spraying the parchment with cooking spray.

2. Using the prepared baking sheet, evenly distribute the nuts. Bake until aromatic, 8 to 10 minutes. Take them out of the oven and leave it on while they cool somewhat.

3. In a small bowl, mix together lemon zest, lemon juice, honey, Berbere, and Aleppo pepper.

4. Transfer the nuts to a large bowl and pour the honey-spice mixture over them. Toss to coat evenly.

5. Return the nut mixture to the baking sheet, spreading it into an even layer. Bake for an additional 8 to 10 minutes until the nuts are caramelized.

6. Remove from the oven and let them cool completely before serving.

Nutrition: Calories: 336; Fat: 7g; Carbs: 17g; Protein: 11g

6. Walnut-Garlic Yogurt Dip

Preparation time: 10 minutes

Cooking time: 0 minutes

Servings: 4

Ingredients:

- 2 cups plain low-fat yogurt

- 3 garlic cloves, minced

- ¼ cup dill, chopped

- 1 green onion, chopped

- ¼ cup walnuts, chopped

- Salt & black pepper to taste

Directions:

1. Combine garlic, yogurt, dill, walnuts, salt, and pepper in a bowl.

2. Serve topped with green onion.

Nutrition: Calories: 210; Fat: 7g; Carbs: 16g; Protein: 9g

7. Oven-Baked Potato Wedges

Preparation time: 10 minutes

Cooking time: 40 minutes

Servings: 4

Ingredients:

- 2 tbsp olive oil

- 4 potatoes, cut into wedges

- 2 tbsp grated Parmesan cheese

- Salt & black pepper to taste

Directions:

1. Preheat the oven to 340°F.

2. In a bowl, toss the potatoes with olive oil, salt, and black pepper. Spread them on a lined baking sheet and bake for 40 minutes until the edges are golden brown.

3. Serve the crispy wedges sprinkled with Parmesan cheese.

Nutrition: Calories: 359; Fat: 8g; Carbs: 66g; Protein: 9g

8. Mediterranean Artichoke Antipasto

Preparation time: 10 minutes

Cooking time: 0 minutes

Servings: 4

Ingredients:

- 1 jar roasted red peppers

- 8 canned artichoke hearts

- 1 can garbanzo beans

- 1 cup whole Kalamata olives

- ¼ cup balsamic vinegar

- Salt to taste

- Zest of 1 lemon

Directions:

1. Slice the roasted red peppers and place them in a large bowl. Quarter the canned artichoke hearts and add them to the bowl.

2. Include the garbanzo beans, Kalamata olives, balsamic vinegar, lemon zest, and salt. Toss all the ingredients together. Serve the antipasto chilled.

Nutrition: Calories: 281; Fat: 15g; Carbs: 30g; Protein: 7g

9. Roasted Sweet Potato Hummus

Preparation time: 10 minutes

Cooking time: 60 minutes

Servings: 8-10

Ingredients:

- 1 lb. sweet potatoes

- 1 (15-oz) can chickpeas, drained

- 4 garlic cloves, minced

- 2 tbsp olive oil

- 2 tbsp fresh lemon juice

- 2 tsp ground cumin

- 1 tsp Aleppo pepper or red pepper flakes

- Pita chips, pita bread, or fresh vegetables, for serving

Directions:

1. Preheat the oven to 400ºF.

2. Prick the sweet potatoes in a few places with a small, sharp knife and place them on a baking sheet.

3. Roast until cooked through, about 1 hour, then set aside to cool. Peel the sweet potatoes and put the flesh in a blender or food processor.

4. Add the chickpeas, garlic, olive oil, lemon juice, cumin, and 1/3 cup water. Blend until smooth. Add the Aleppo pepper. Serve with pita chips, pita bread, or as a dip for fresh vegetables.

Nutrition: Calories: 178; Fat: 5g; Carbs: 30g; Protein: 7g

10. Manchego Cheese Crackers

Preparation time: 10 minutes

Cooking time: 15 minutes

Servings: 40 crackers

Ingredients:

- 4 tbsp butter, at room temperature

- 1 cup finely shredded Manchego cheese

- 1 cup almond flour

- 1 tsp salt, divided

- ¼ tsp freshly ground black pepper

- 1 large egg

Directions:

1. Using an electric mixer, cream together the butter and shredded cheese until well combined and smooth.

2. In a small bowl, combine the almond flour with ½ teaspoon salt and pepper.

3. Slowly add the almond flour mixture to the cheese, mixing constantly until the dough just comes together to form a ball.

4. Transfer to a piece of parchment or plastic wrap and roll into a cylinder log about 1½ inches thick. Refrigerate for a minimum of one hour after securely wrapping.

5. Preheat the oven to 350ºF, and line two baking sheets with parchment paper or silicone baking mats.

6. To make the egg wash, in a small bowl, whisk the egg and remaining ½ teaspoon salt.

7. Slice the refrigerated dough into small rounds, about ¼ inch thick, and place on the lined baking sheets.

8. Bake the crackers for 12 to 15 minutes, or until they are golden and crispy, after brushing the tops with egg wash. Take out of the oven and place on a wire rack to cool. Warm up and serve.

Nutrition: Calories: 73; Fat: 7g; Carbs: 1g; Protein: 3g

1. Almond Butter Cup Fat Bomb

Prep time: 10 minutes

Cooking time: 0 minutes

Servings: 8

Ingredients

- ½ cup crunchy almond butter (no sugar added)

- ½ cup light fruity extra-virgin olive oil

- ¼ cup ground flaxseed

- 2 tbsp unsweetened cocoa powder

- 1 tsp vanilla extract

- 1 tsp ground cinnamon (optional)

- 1 to 2 tsp sugar-free sweetener of choice (optional)

Directions:

1. In a mixing bowl, combine the almond butter, olive oil, flaxseed, cocoa powder, vanilla, cinnamon (if using), and sweetener (if using) and stir well with a spatula to combine.

2. Pour into 8 mini muffin liners and freeze until solid, at least 12 hours. Store in the freezer to maintain their shape.

Nutrition: Calories: 239; Fat: 4g; Carbs: 5g; Protein: 4g

2. Strawberry Panna Cotta

Preparation time: 10 minutes + chilling time

Cooking time: 0 minutes

Servings: 4

Ingredients:

- 2 tbsp warm water

- 2 tsp gelatin powder

- 2 cups heavy cream

- 1 cup sliced strawberries, plus more for garnish

- 1 to 2 tbsp sugar-free sweetener of choice (optional)

- 1½ tsp pure vanilla extract

- 4 to 6 fresh mint leaves, for garnish (optional)

Directions:

1. Pour the warm water into a small bowl. Sprinkle the gelatin over the water and stir well to dissolve. Allow the mixture to sit for 10 minutes.

2. In a blender or a large bowl, if using an immersion blender, combine the cream, strawberries, sweetener (if using), and vanilla.

3. Blend until the mixture is smooth and the strawberries are well puréed. Transfer the mixture to a saucepan and heat over medium-low heat until just below a simmer.

4. Remove from the heat and cool for 5 minutes. Whisking constantly, add in the gelatin mixture until smooth.

5. Divide the custard between ramekins or small glass bowls, cover and refrigerate until set, 4 to 6 hours.

6. Serve chilled, garnishing with additional sliced strawberries or mint leaves (if using).

Nutrition: Calories: 229; Fat: 12g; Carbs: 5g; Protein: 3g

3. Orange–Olive Oil Cupcakes

Preparation time: 10 minutes

Cooking time: 18 minutes

Servings: 6 cupcakes

Ingredients:

- 1 large egg

- 2 tbsp powdered sugar-free sweetener

- ½ cup extra-virgin olive oil

- 1 tsp almond extract

- Zest of 1 orange

- 1 cup almond flour

- ¾ tsp baking powder

- 1/8 tsp salt

- 1 tbsp freshly squeezed orange juice

Directions:

1. Preheat the oven to 350°F, and place muffin liners into 6 cups of a muffin tin.

2. In a large bowl, whisk together the egg and powdered sweetener. Add the olive oil, almond extract, and orange zest and whisk to combine well.

3. In a small bowl, whisk together the almond flour, baking powder, and salt. Add to wet ingredients along with the orange juice and stir until just combined.

4. Evenly divide the batter among 6 muffin cups. Bake for 15 to 18 minutes, or until a toothpick inserted in the center of a cupcake comes out clean.

5. Remove from the oven and cool for 5 minutes in the tin before transferring to a wire rack to cool completely.

Nutrition: Calories: 28; Fat: 7g; Carbs: 8g; Protein: 4g

4. Olive Oil Ice Cream

Preparation time: 10 minutes + freezing time

Cooking time: 25 minutes

Servings: 8

Ingredients:

- 4 large egg yolks

- 1/3 cup powdered sugar-free sweetener

- 2 cups half-and-half

- 1 tsp vanilla extract

- 1/8 tsp salt

- ¼ cup light fruity extra-virgin olive oil

Directions:

1. Freeze the bowl of an ice cream maker for at least 12 hours or overnight.

2. In a large bowl, whisk together the egg yolks and sugar-free sweetener.

3. In a small saucepan, heat the half-and-half over medium heat until just below a boil. Take off the heat source and let it cool down a little.

4. To prevent the eggs from cooking, gradually add the heated half-and-half to the egg mixture while whisking continuously. Place the saucepan back on low heat and add the eggs and cream.

5. Cook over low heat, whisking continually, until thickened, 15 to 20 minutes. Take off the heat and mix in the salt and vanilla essence.

6. Transfer to a glass bowl after whisking in the olive oil. Let cool, cover, and chill for a minimum of six hours. In an ice cream machine, freeze custard as directed by the manufacturer.

Nutrition: Calories: 168; Fat: 5g; Carbs: 8g; Protein: 2g

5. Pumpkin-Ricotta Cheesecake

Preparation time: 15 minutes

Cooking time: 45 minutes

Servings: 10-12

Ingredients:

- 1 cup almond flour

- ½ cup melted butter

- 1 (14½-oz) can pumpkin purée

- 8 oz cream cheese, at room temperature

- ½ cup whole-milk ricotta cheese

- ½ to ¾ cup sugar-free sweetener

- 4 large eggs

- 2 tsp vanilla extract

- 2 tsp pumpkin pie spice

- Whipped cream, for garnish (optional)

Directions:

1. Preheat the oven to 350ºF, and line the bottom of a 9-inch spring form pan with parchment paper.

2. In a small bowl, combine the almond flour and melted butter with a fork until well combined. Using your fingers, press the mixture into the bottom of the prepared pan.

3. In a large bowl, beat together the pumpkin purée, cream cheese, ricotta, and sweetener using an electric mixer on medium.

4. Add the eggs, one at a time, beating after each addition. Stir in the vanilla and pumpkin pie spice until just combined.

5. Pour the mixture over the crust and bake until set, 40 to 45 minutes. Allow to cool to room temperature.

6. Before serving, place in the fridge for at least six hours. If preferred, top with whipped cream and serve chilled.

Nutrition: Calories: 230; Fat: 11g; Carbs: 5g; Protein: 6g

6. Grilled Stone Fruit with Whipped Ricotta

Preparation time: 10 minutes

Cooking time: 10 minutes

Servings: 4

Ingredients:

- Nonstick cooking spray

- 4 peaches or nectarines, halved & pitted

- 2 tsp extra-virgin olive oil

- ¾ cup whole-milk ricotta cheese

- 1 tbsp honey

- ¼ tsp freshly grated nutmeg

- 4 sprigs mint, for garnish (optional)

Directions:

1. Apply nonstick cooking spray to a grill pan or cold grill. Turn up the heat to medium on the grill or grill pan. To chill, put a large, empty bowl in the fridge.

2. Brush the fruit all over with the oil. Place the fruit cut-side down on the grill or pan and cook for 3 to 5 minutes, or until grill marks appear.

3. Using tongs, turn the fruit over. Cover the grill and cook for 4 to 6 minutes, until the fruit is easily pierced with a sharp knife. Set aside to cool.

4. Remove the bowl from the refrigerator and add the ricotta. Using an electric beater, beat the ricotta on high for 2 minutes.

5. Add the honey and nutmeg and beat for 1 more minute.

6. Divide the warm (or room temperature) fruit among 4 serving bowls, top with the ricotta mixture, and a sprig of mint (if using) and serve.

Nutrition: Calories: 180; Fat: 9g; Carbs: 21g; Protein: 7g

7. Chocolate-Dipped Fruit Bites

Preparation time: 10 minutes

Cooking time: 0 minutes

Servings: 4-6

Ingredients:

- ½ cup semisweet chocolate chips

- ¼ cup low-fat milk

- ½ tsp pure vanilla extract

- ½ tsp ground nutmeg

- ¼ tsp salt

- 2 kiwis, peeled and sliced

- 1 cup honeydew melon chunks

- 1 lb. whole strawberries

Directions:

1. Place the chocolate chips in a small bowl.

2. In another small bowl, microwave the milk until hot, about 30 seconds.

3. Pour the milk over the chocolate chips and let sit for 1 minute, then whisk until the chocolate is melted and smooth.

4. Stir in the vanilla, nutmeg, and salt and allow to cool for 5 minutes. Line a baking sheet with wax paper.

5. Dip each piece of fruit halfway into the chocolate, tap gently to remove excess chocolate, and place the fruit on the baking sheet.

6. Once all the fruit has been dipped, allow it to sit until dry, about 30 minutes. Arrange on a platter and serve.

Nutrition: Calories: 125; Fat: 5g; Carbs: 21g; Protein: 2g

8. Almond Cocoa Bites

Preparation time: 10 minutes

Cooking time: 0 minutes

Servings: 6

Ingredients:

- ½ cup roasted, unsalted whole almonds (with skins)

- 3 tbsp granulated sugar, divided

- 1½ tsp unsweetened cocoa powder

- 1¼ tbsp unseasoned breadcrumbs

- ¾ tsp pure vanilla extract

- 1½ tsp orange juice

Directions:

1. Place the almonds in a food processor and process until you have a coarse ground texture.

2. In a medium bowl, combine the ground almonds, 2 tablespoons sugar, the cocoa powder, and the breadcrumbs. Mix well.

3. In a small bowl, combine the vanilla extract and orange juice. Stir and then add the mixture to the almond mixture. Mix well.

4. Measure out a teaspoon of the mixture. Squeeze the mixture with your hand to make the dough stick together, then mold the dough into a small ball.

5. Add the remaining tablespoon of sugar to a shallow bowl. Roll the balls in the sugar until covered, then transfer the bites to an airtight container. Serve.

Nutrition: Calories: 102; Fat: 6g; Carbs: 10g; Protein: 3g

9. Ricotta with Balsamic Cherries and Black Pepper

Preparation time: 10 minutes

Cooking time: 0 minutes

Servings: 4

Ingredients:

- 1 cup ricotta

- 2 tbsp honey

- 1 tsp vanilla extract

- 3 cups pitted sweet cherries (thawed if frozen), halved

- 1½ tsp aged balsamic vinegar

- Pinch of freshly ground black pepper

Directions

1. Place the ricotta, honey, and vanilla in a food processor and mix until smooth. After moving the mixture to a medium-sized bowl, cover it, and chill it for a full hour.

2. In a small bowl, combine the cherries, vinegar, and pepper and stir to mix well. Chill along with the ricotta mixture.

3. To serve, spoon the ricotta mixture into 4 serving bowls or glasses.

4. Top with the cherries, dividing them equally and spooning a bit of the accumulated juice over the top of each bowl. Serve chilled.

Nutrition: Calories: 236; Fat: 5g; Carbs: 42g; Protein: 7g

10. Date and Honey Almond Milk Ice Cream

Preparation time: 10 minutes + freezing time

Cooking time: 5 minutes

Servings: 4

Ingredients:

- ¾ cup pitted dates

- ¼ cup honey

- ½ cup water

- 2 cups cold unsweetened almond milk

- 2 tsp vanilla extract

Directions:

1. Combine the dates and water in a small saucepan and bring to a boil over high heat. Remove the pan from the heat, cover, and let stand for 15 minutes.

2. In a blender, combine the almond milk, dates, the date soaking water, honey, and the vanilla and process until very smooth.

3. Cover the blender jar and refrigerate the mixture until cold, at least 1 hour.

4. Transfer the mixture to an electric ice cream maker and freeze according to the manufacturer's instructions.

5. Serve immediately or transfer to a freezer-safe storage container and freeze for 4 hours (or longer). Serve frozen.

Nutrition: Calories: 106; Fat: 2g; Carbs: 23g; Protein: 1g

28-day meal plan

Breakfast:

Tomato Scrambled Eggs

Lunch:

Pesto-Glazed Chicken Breasts

Dinner:

Bruschetta Chicken Burgers

Salad:

Zesty Feta and Olive Blend

Legumes, Grains, and Pasta:

Bucatini in Puttanesca Style

Snack and Appetizers:

Hummus-Cucumber Delight

Dessert:

Almond Butter Cup Fat Bomb

Day 2:

Breakfast:

Morning Baklava French Toast

Lunch:

Arugula Spinach Salad with Shaved Parmesan

Dinner:

Classic Margherita Pizza

Salad:

Garlic-infused Broccoli Rabe with Artichokes

Legumes, Grains, and Pasta:

White Bean Lettuce Wraps

Snack and Appetizers:

Feta and Artichoke Medley

Dessert:

Strawberry Panna Cotta

Day 3:

Breakfast:

Buckwheat Porridge

Lunch:

Shrimp Quinoa Bowl with Black Olives

Dinner:

Pistachio-Crusted Baked Fish

Salad:

Greens Braised with Olives and Walnuts

Legumes, Grains, and Pasta:

Mango Infused Chili Black Beans

Snack and Appetizers:

Maple-Spiced Nut Medley

Dessert:

Orange–Olive Oil Cupcakes

Day 4:

Breakfast:

Egg in a "Pepper Hole" with Avocado

Lunch:

Margherita Open-Face Sandwiches

Dinner:

Bomba Chicken with Chickpeas

Salad:

Roasted Honey Acorn Squash

Legumes, Grains, and Pasta:

Fava Bean and Garbanzo Fūl

Snack and Appetizers:

Arugula Pesto Dip

Dessert:

Olive Oil Ice Cream

Day 5:

Breakfast:

Avocado Toast with Smoked Trout

Lunch:

Zucchini with Bow Ties

Dinner:

Ratatouille

Salad:

Oven-Baked Beet and Leek with Dilly Yogurt

Legumes, Grains, and Pasta:

Halloumi and Green Bean Salad

Snack and Appetizers:

Citrus-Spiced Nut Mix

Dessert:

Pumpkin-Ricotta Cheesecake

Day 6:

Breakfast:

Kale Egg Cups

Lunch:

Pan-Fried Chili Sea Scallops

Dinner:

Pork Chops in Tomato Olive Sauce

Salad:

Wok-Style Kale with Mushrooms

Legumes, Grains, and Pasta:

Tuscan-Style Baked Beans

Snack and Appetizers:

Walnut-Garlic Yogurt Dip

Dessert:

Grilled Stone Fruit with Whipped Ricotta

Day 7:

Breakfast:

Banana Pancakes With

Lunch:

Herb–Marinated Chicken Breasts

Dinner:

Olive & Escarole Salmon

Salad:

Zesty Zucchini Cubes with Mint

Legumes, Grains, and Pasta:

Pinto Bean Salad

Snack and Appetizers:

Oven-Baked Potato Wedges

Dessert:

Chocolate-Dipped Fruit Bites

Day 8:

Breakfast:

Pecan & Peach Parfait

Lunch:

Dill Salmon Salad Wraps

Dinner:

Moroccan Lamb Wrap with Harissa

Salad:

Herbed Marinated Mushrooms and Olives

Legumes, Grains, and Pasta:

Golden Organic Chickpeas

Snack and Appetizers:

Mediterranean Artichoke Antipasto

Dessert:

Almond Cocoa Bites

Day 9:

Breakfast:

Breakfast Pita Sandwiches

Lunch:

Hake Fillet in Herby Tomato Sauce

Dinner:

Baked Falafel Sliders

Salad:

Parmesan Roasted Cauliflower and Tomatoes

Legumes, Grains, and Pasta:

Yogurt and Chickpea Delight

Snack and Appetizers:

Manchego Cheese Crackers

Dessert:

Ricotta with Balsamic Cherries and Black Pepper

Day 10:

Breakfast:

Chia & Almond Oatmeal

Lunch:

Orzo-Stuffed Tomatoes

Dinner:

Spicy Tomato and Caper Squid Stew

Salad:

Legumes, Grains, and Pasta: Parmesan Roasted Cauliflower and Tomatoes

Snack and Appetizers:

Maple-Spiced Nut Medley

Dessert:

Date and Honey Almond Milk Ice Cream

Day 11:

Breakfast:

Breakfast Bulgur with Berries

Lunch:

Sautéed Lemon & Garlic Chicken

Dinner:

Harissa Yogurt Chicken Thighs

Salad:

Zesty Feta and Olive Blend

Legumes, Grains, and Pasta:

Bucatini in Puttanesca Style

Snack and Appetizers:

Hummus-Cucumber Delight

Dessert:

Almond Butter Cup Fat Bomb

Day 12:

Breakfast:

Strawberry Basil Honey Ricotta Toast

Lunch:

Quick Shrimp Fettuccine

Dinner:

Baked Asparagus Caprese Pasta

Salad:

Garlic-infused Broccoli Rabe with Artichokes

Legumes, Grains, and Pasta:

White Bean Lettuce Wraps

Snack and Appetizers:

Feta and Artichoke Medley

Dessert:

Strawberry Panna Cotta

Day 13:

Breakfast:

Parsley Tomato Eggs

Lunch:

Tender Pork Shoulder

Dinner:

Lemon Trout with Roasted Beets

Salad:

Oven-Baked Beet and Leek with Dilly Yogurt

Legumes, Grains, and Pasta:

Mango Infused Chili Black Beans

Snack and Appetizers:

Maple-Spiced Nut Medley

Dessert:

Orange–Olive Oil Cupcakes

Day 14:

Breakfast:

Garlic Bell Pepper Omelet

Lunch:

Grilled Eggplant and Feta Sandwiches

Dinner:

Date Lamb Tagine

Salad:

Zesty Zucchini Cubes with Mint

Legumes, Grains, and Pasta:

Halloumi and Green Bean Salad

Snack and Appetizers:

Citrus-Spiced Nut Mix

Conclusion

In conclusion, the Cirrhosis Liver Cookbook aims to provide not just a collection of delicious recipes but also a thoughtful guide for individuals managing cirrhosis. Navigating dietary choices can be a crucial aspect of maintaining liver health, and this cookbook seeks to offer a diverse range of flavorful and nutrient-rich meals.

The recipes included emphasize the use of ingredients known for their liver-friendly properties while maintaining a focus on taste and enjoyment. It is essential to consult with healthcare professionals for personalized advice, but the recipes presented here can serve as a starting point for those seeking flavorful and nourishing options.

Whether you're looking for breakfast ideas, lunch and dinner inspirations, refreshing salads, legume-centric dishes, or delightful desserts, the cookbook aspires to support individuals on their journey toward better liver health. Remember, every meal is an opportunity to nourish the body and savor the pleasure of eating, even when managing specific health conditions.

Wishing you good health and culinary joy on your path to wellness!

Happy cooking!!!

1. **What is cirrhosis of the liver?**

    - Cirrhosis is a late stage of scarring (fibrosis) of the liver caused by many forms of liver diseases and conditions, such as hepatitis and chronic alcoholism.

2. **What are the common causes of cirrhosis?**

    - Cirrhosis can result from various factors, including chronic alcoholism, viral hepatitis (B, C, D), nonalcoholic fatty liver disease (NAFLD), and autoimmune liver diseases.

3. **What are the symptoms of cirrhosis?**

    - Symptoms may include fatigue, weakness, easy bruising, swelling in the legs and abdomen, confusion, and jaundice (yellowing of the skin and eyes).

4. **How is cirrhosis diagnosed?**

    - Diagnosis often involves a combination of medical history, physical examination, blood tests, imaging studies (ultrasound, CT scan), and sometimes a liver biopsy.

5. **Can cirrhosis be reversed?**

    - In the early stages, lifestyle changes and treating the underlying cause may slow or stop the progression of cirrhosis. However, once extensive scarring occurs, it is usually irreversible.

6. **What dietary considerations are important for individuals with cirrhosis?**

- A balanced diet with reduced sodium intake is crucial. Monitoring protein, managing fluid intake, and avoiding alcohol are also key dietary considerations.

7. **Is exercise recommended for individuals with cirrhosis?**

   - Moderate exercise can be beneficial, but it's important to consult with healthcare professionals to determine an appropriate exercise plan based on individual health status.

8. **Can cirrhosis lead to liver cancer?**

   - Yes, cirrhosis increases the risk of liver cancer (hepatocellular carcinoma). Regular monitoring and screenings are essential for early detection.

9. **How can complications like ascites and varices be managed?**

   - Medications, dietary changes, and in some cases, medical procedures may be recommended to manage complications like ascites (fluid buildup) and varices (enlarged blood vessels).

10. **What support is available for individuals with cirrhosis?**

    - Support groups, counseling, and education from healthcare providers play a crucial role. Social and emotional support is essential for individuals and their caregivers.

Meal Planner
Journal

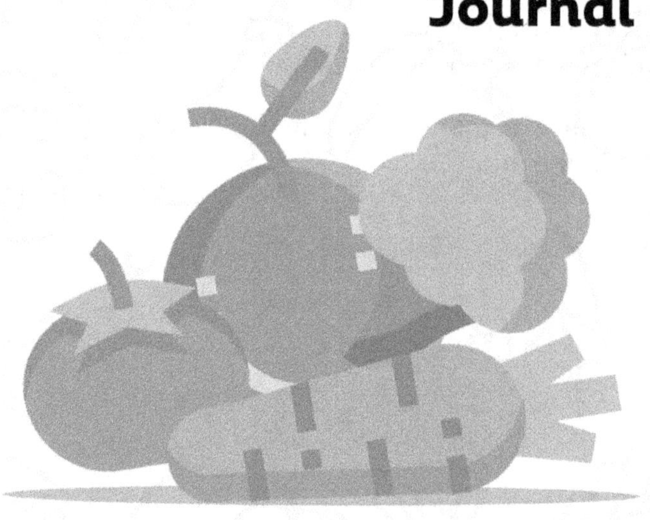

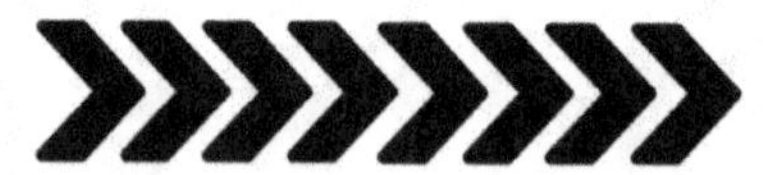

S M T W T F S

WATER

MENU LIST:

Breakfast:

Lunch:

Dinner:

Shopping list:

Important Meal:

To-do List:

Note and Tips:

EAT HEALTHY

MENU LIST:

Breakfast:

Lunch:

Dinner:

Shopping list:

Important Meal:

To-do List:

Note and Tips:

MENU LIST:

Breakfast:

Lunch:

Dinner:

Important Meal:

To-do List:

Shopping list:

Note and Tips:

S M T W T F S
○ ○ ○ ○ ○ ○ ○

WATER
○ ○ ○ ○ ○ ○ ○

MENU LIST:

Breakfast:

Lunch:

Dinner:

Important Meal:

To-do List:

Shopping list:

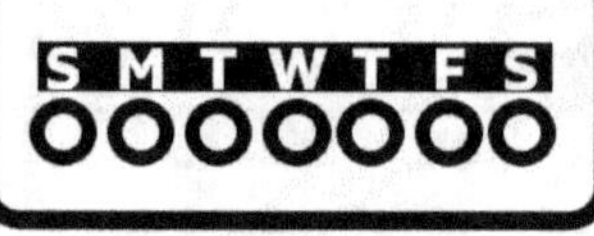

Note and Tips:

S M T W T F S
○ ○ ○ ○ ○ ○ ○

WATER
○ ○ ○ ○ ○ ○ ○

MENU LIST:

Breakfast:

Lunch:

Dinner:

Shopping list:
____
____
____
____

Important Meal:

To-do List:
____
____
____

Note and Tips:

MENU LIST:

Breakfast:

Lunch:

Dinner:

Important Meal:

To-do List:

Shopping list:

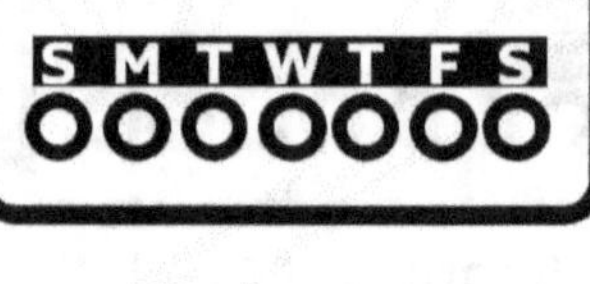

Note and Tips:

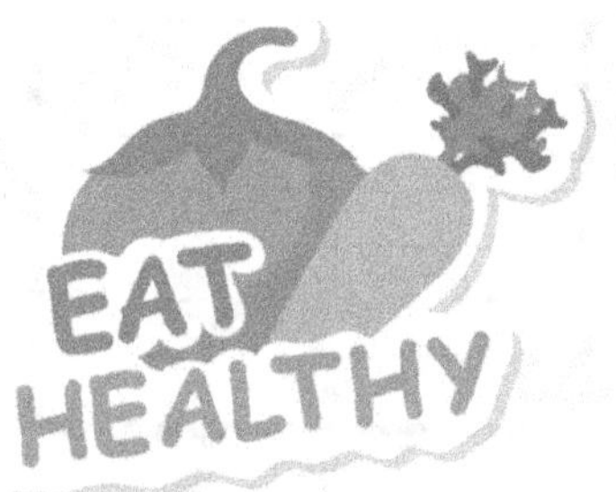

MENU LIST:

Breakfast:

Lunch:

Dinner:

Important Meal:

Shopping list:

To-do List:

Note and Tips:

MENU LIST:

Breakfast:

Lunch:

Dinner:

Important Meal:

To-do List:

Shopping list:

Note and Tips:

MENU LIST:

Breakfast:

Lunch:

Dinner:

Shopping list:

Important Meal:

To-do List:

Note and Tips:

S M T W T F S

WATER

MENU LIST:

Breakfast:

Lunch:

Dinner:

Important Meal:

To-do List:

Shopping list:

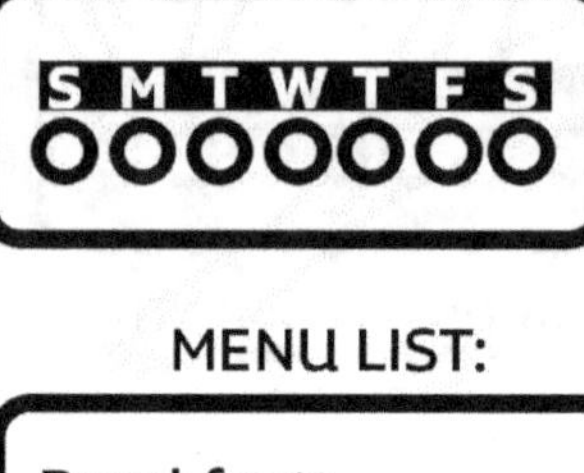

Note and Tips:

MENU LIST:

Breakfast:

Lunch:

Dinner:

Important Meal:

To-do List:

Shopping list:

Note and Tips:

MENU LIST:

Breakfast:

Lunch:

Dinner:

Important Meal:

To-do List:

Shopping list:

Note and Tips:

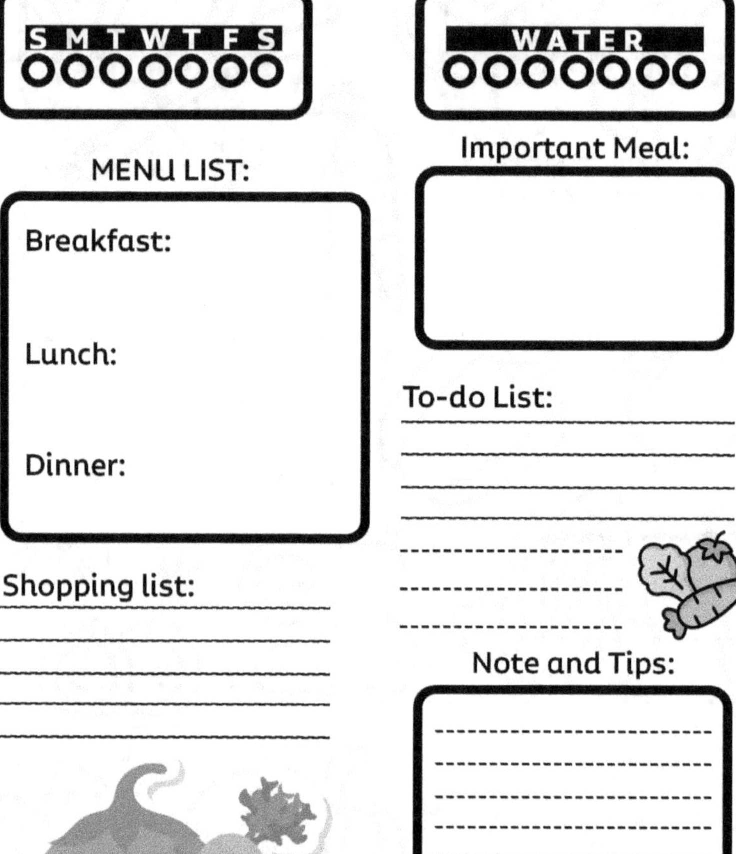

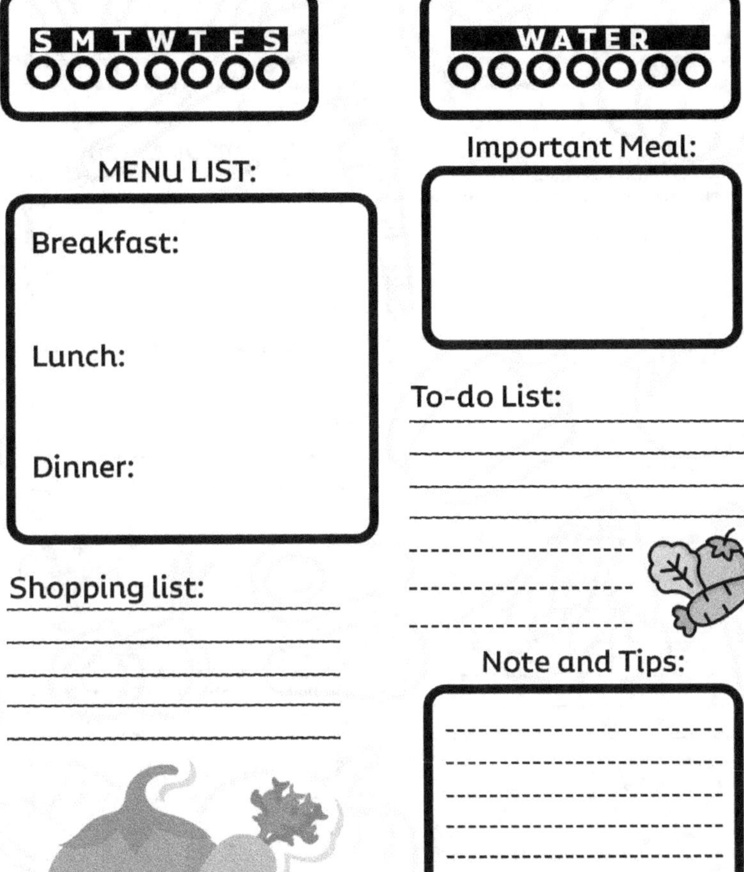

S M T W T F S

WATER

MENU LIST:

Breakfast:

Lunch:

Dinner:

Important Meal:

To-do List:

Shopping list:

Note and Tips:

EAT HEALTHY

MENU LIST:

Breakfast:

Lunch:

Dinner:

Important Meal:

To-do List:

Shopping list:

Note and Tips:

MENU LIST:

Breakfast:

Lunch:

Dinner:

Important Meal:

To-do List:

Shopping list:

Note and Tips:

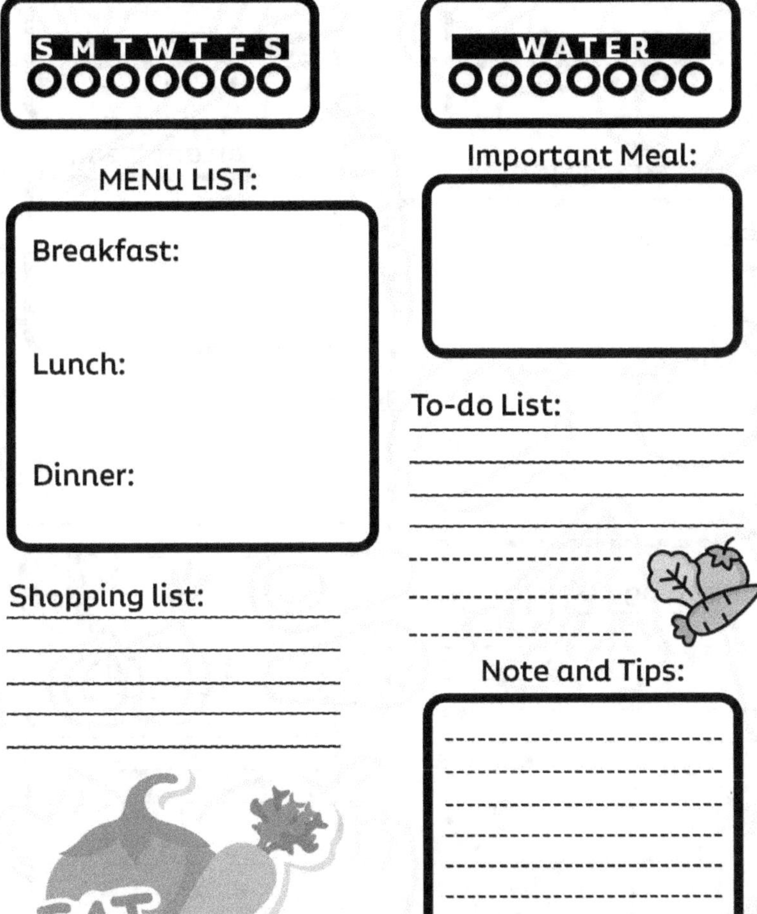

MENU LIST:

Breakfast:

Lunch:

Dinner:

Important Meal:

Shopping list:

To-do List:

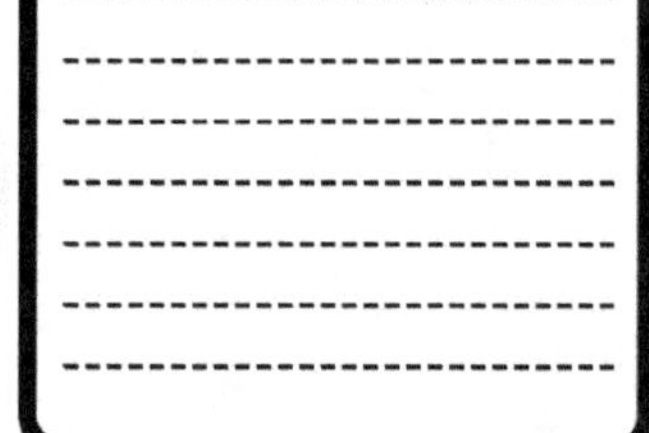

Note and Tips:

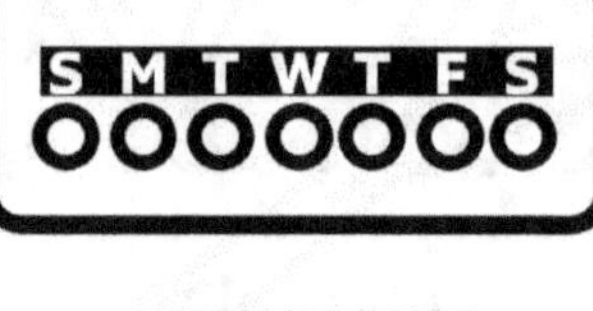

MENU LIST:

Breakfast:

Lunch:

Dinner:

Shopping list:

Important Meal:

To-do List:

Note and Tips:

MENU LIST:

Breakfast:

Lunch:

Dinner:

Important Meal:

To-do List:

Shopping list:

Note and Tips:

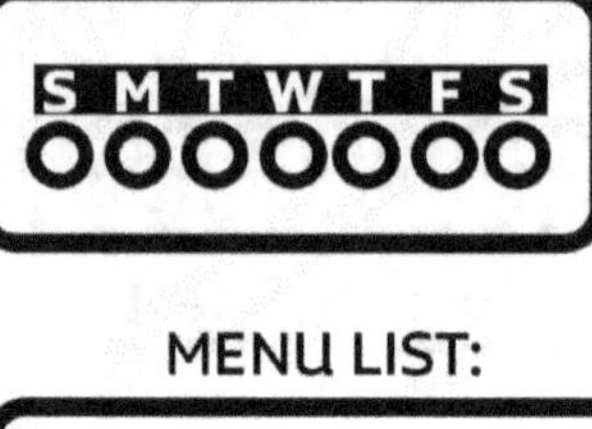

MENU LIST:

Breakfast:

Lunch:

Dinner:

Important Meal:

To-do List:

Shopping list:

Note and Tips:

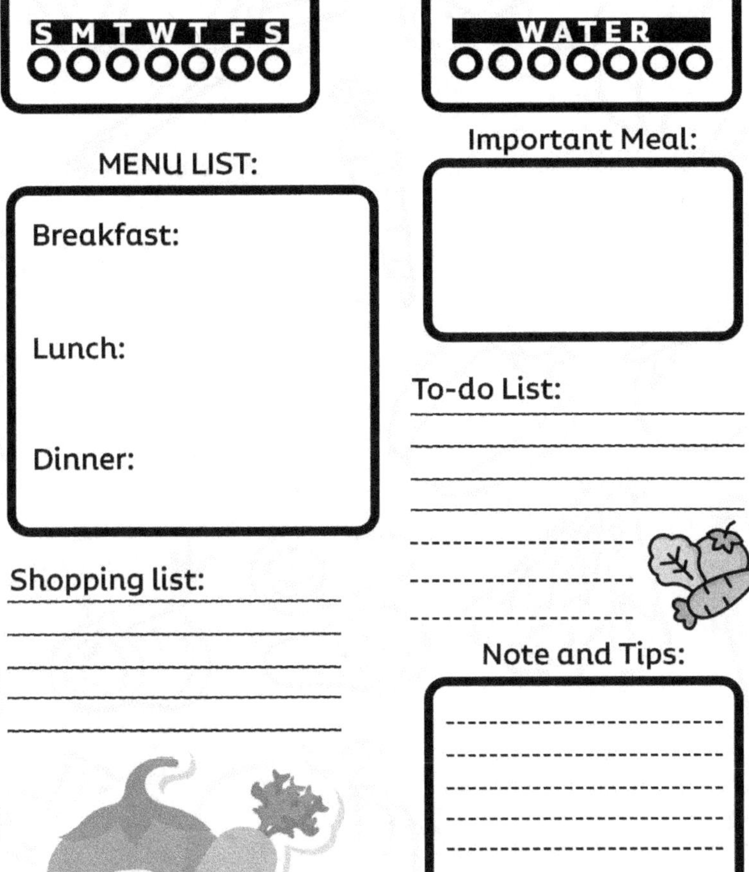